Rachel McGrath grew up in Redcliffe, a seaside town in Queensland, Australia, where she studied Business, before moving to the United Kingdom in her early thirties. She currently lives just north of London, where she met and married her husband. She has a professional career in human resources. Rachel has always had a passion for writing both fiction and non-fiction, creating many short stories from her early teens as well as smaller pieces of work that have never been published. *Finding the Rainbow* is Rachel's first novel, a story capturing a difficult time in her life; she is passionate about sharing this with a wider audience.

Finding the Rainbow was awarded the People's Book Prize winner in 2016, and was also a Bronze medal winner in the Reader's Favorite awards. Rachel has a strong following all over the world via her personal blog www.findingthrainbow.net

Rachel McGrath

Finding the Rainbow

McGrath House

McGRATH HOUSE PAPERBACK

© Copyright 2017
2nd Edition
Rachel McGrath

A CIP catalogue record for this title is
available from the British Library.

Although the author and publisher have made every effort to ensure that the
information in this book was correct at press time, the author and publisher do not
assume and hereby disclaim any liability to any party for any loss, damage, or
disruption caused by errors or omissions, whether such errors or omissions result
from negligence, accident, or any other cause.

ISBN 978-1542494557

**First edition Published in 2015 by Vanguard Press
Second edition 2017 by McGrath House**

This book is dedicated to my husband: my partner, soul mate and best friend. We have been on this journey together, working through some of the toughest moments a couple can experience. He is my rock, always there to hold my hand and keep me positive.

A brief word before we start

To all the mums and dads, and the hopeful mums and dads to be, this is not a reference book, and nor is it meant to be. It's not a guide on how to fall pregnant and stay pregnant, and it certainly won't take you through each and every exciting month of pregnancy with tips and techniques on your health, wellbeing and growing baby.

This story is purely an account of my own experience when trying to conceive. Something I put pen to paper, to help reconcile what I went through, to manage my feelings and internal thoughts through a period that has been a crazy, rollercoaster ride of emotions. Trying for a baby was both a mental and physical journey of excitement, hope and loss, something I had never imagined would be so difficult and sometimes so painful.

Whether you are thinking about getting pregnant, trying to conceive, are in the midst of your pregnancy, or you are fortunate to be holding that bundle of joy, you will understand that each and every couple has a very different experience. I found that my experiences even differed throughout each of my pregnancies. Unfortunately there is no set formula, rhyme or reason when it comes to falling pregnant, or starting a family and that really is the beauty and the pain of this amazing journey.

This is my journey through early pregnancy: the good the bad and the ugly. This is my personal account of how I felt, what I experienced, the highs and the lows, and sometimes how I dealt with the setbacks I was forced to face on our baby-making road.

I do not wish to advocate any advice throughout this story, or provide any false hopes or crush any dreams. I wrote this to share my experience of a personal topic that many women don't seem to talk openly about.

It was something I realised during my pregnancies and my losses. Many women and men see the subject of early pregnancy loss as taboo, and generally avoid discussing their own experiences. Perhaps it is too hard and too painful to discuss, perhaps it's the knowledge that others will be questioning them on what happened, or what they will do next. I'm not really sure.

Many couples we know didn't tell a soul that they had experienced infertility, loss and disappointment in the early stages of pregnancy. Most, I found, would wait until the end of the first trimester, or even late into the second trimester before sharing their exciting news with close family and friends that they were even expecting. It was a nice little secret most couples kept to themselves in those earlier days of pregnancy. During those exciting times when we found out we were pregnant, I suppose keeping it between myself and my husband would have been something just for us to know, and enjoy that moment. However, I guess I'm a little different to the norm, and it's probably why you're reading this now.

What I found is that each time I went through the process of excitement to apprehension and loss, it was the support from friends and family that helped me stay strong. My workplace was supportive and understanding and it really wasn't worth the time and effort for me to be secretive about what I had gone through. Especially with the number of hospital and doctor's appointments I ended up attending.

However, in saying this, I appreciate that this was the way I coped with my personal feelings and experiences, and that everyone has different needs and therefore may approach things very differently. There is no right or wrong way to manage pregnancy and loss, there is only your own way.

I hope that my story is helpful in some way.

New Horizons

The world of 'trying to conceive' is a place that is both physically, mentally and emotionally all consuming. It's a place I didn't even know existed until two years ago and frankly one I was quite unprepared for.

At the age of thirty-six, I had no idea of the impact of cycle times or when I actually ovulated, and then there were Basel temperatures, cervical mucus, days past ovulation, implantation and the hope of that elusive 'Big Fat Positive' result! Many couples at certain points in their life or at various ages make that important decision to start a family, and this then starts a cycle for some that results in a very quick positive result and a lovely bundle of joy! For others, it's a tough road filled with hope, heartbreak and turmoil, with numerous unsuccessful conception cycles and early pregnancy loss through miscarriage. So how do you really prepare for this?

I'm not sure you can. Whilst I possibly didn't really understand the world of trying to conceive, you quickly learn as you enter it. I recall discussing with my husband how we would probably be pregnant within the first couple of months. We were so excited! We were very naïve. Many people had warned me, saying I would have a challenge being 'over thirty-five years', but we were both fit and healthy with an active sex life, so why would we have any problems?

I had a number of friends who had prior miscarriages or fertility problems, and again that hadn't phased me. Of course I'm different, and it will happen for us, I'd thought. We will have a family within the next twelve months. I was so certain of that.

It was seven months before I got my first positive pregnancy result. I was getting incredibly frustrated at that point, thinking it would never happen, and that there was actually something really wrong. We even started to look at alternative options like adoption or surrogacy. A little premature, but that's me all over; I'm impatient. If you were to compare my experience with others, seven months is actually a good result. I had heard of many others who had tried for over twelve months before getting pregnant the first time.

Whilst we didn't have a first successful pregnancy, it gave us hope. That's just part of the story that you will read in the later chapters. What I found is that pregnancy is a journey, with many bumps along the road. The timing of cycles and waiting for results, the hope and excitement of finding out you're pregnant, and then the pain and grief of miscarriage, which often leads to starting all over again; it's not an easy ride for any woman or couple to endure. Nonetheless, it's a passage that many couples unfortunately need to pass through to achieve their ultimate goal, a healthy baby, starting a family and becoming parents. It's one of the ultimate life experiences and an aspiration I've personally dreamt about from as far back as I can remember.

Reflections

Somebody asked me once whether I would go back and change things; whether I would alter my path if I had the choice. Would I have started trying to conceive earlier, start a family, had I known that we would have the challenges we faced? It made me think. Would I? If I had a time machine, would we have started earlier, and would I have looked at my priorities differently?

As I reflected on this question I recalled several events throughout my life that made me really think about motherhood. It was during these events that I may have had a choice to prioritise my decisions differently about family and my quest to become a mother.

Looking back, I'm not clear whether it changed the way I viewed my potential to become a mother, but these events certainly stay with me, even today. Perhaps in some ways, they reaffirmed my path?

In the years before I decided on parenthood, I did find that anyone who was currently a parent, or others who had started the process of conception had an opinion on it, and they were quick to share their views. It was clear that of course everyone's own view was the correct one; that we should accept and follow the same set of guidance, and all will be well in the world.

Who would have thought it was all that easy?

What I have learned is that life is not that easy. There is no clear path; no one right way forward, and fate above all will guide our future. At the end of the day, we all roll the dice, and move forward with the hope that we land where we want to be. If we don't, we just keep rolling.

Regrets? I have none. All I have are my reflections, and the knowledge of different paths I could have taken at different stages of my life.

Specialist Advice

In my early twenties I had a serious relationship; I was young and enjoying life, living in a different state away from my hometown, with a promising career ahead of me. Whilst this was my first serious relationship, the guy himself was not someone I could foresee a long lasting future with. In the end we stayed together for around four years, and that was far too long.

During the time I was in this relationship, I was advised that I had an abnormal cervical smear. In the investigations, my gynaecologist did say to me that I had follow on problems from an appendix operation I had when I was sixteen and possible signs of endometriosis. He told me I should consider starting a family earlier rather than later.

In fact his actual advice was, if you don't start trying soon, you may not be able to have a family in later life naturally. I was young, my life was ahead of me, and for me having a baby at that stage of my life, with a partner who was unreliable and more like a child himself, was the last thing on my mind.

It did stick with me however, and there were times when I reflected on the risk I was taking. The bigger risk to me however, was bringing a child into this world when I wasn't ready to be a mother. I didn't have the financial stability to offer a growing child, the structural basics, a loving, stable family or a home with a suitable environment for a growing active child. Finally, I still wanted for things in life, to experience the things I aspired to achieve, personally and professionally. I never wanted regret, and personally it would have been unfair to start a family when I wasn't ready. Had I taken my doctor's advice, that child would be almost fifteen years old, and my life would be very different. The big question to ask is: 'Would I have really regretted starting a family back then?' My perfectly honest answer: 'No'.

As an adult you make life work with the circumstances you are given. I know that any child I might have had at any stage of my life would have been loved wholeheartedly. With one parent or two, with limited financial resources, that child would have had what was necessary and important for a happy healthy life. Love would have been its centre. Nonetheless, I did make a choice at that point in my life, and that choice was with no regrets. I wouldn't be who I am today and we make the decisions in our life for a reason, and life just happens.

Putting My Eggs in One Basket

By the time I was thirty I was single and I had moved interstate again, back to my home city. I had a really good job, I'd bought myself a house, and I was living a fabulous single life with great friends, lots of travels and spending my disposable income on extravagances whilst I could. I actually loved being single and free at this point of my life. I had felt lost in my past relationship, becoming someone I really didn't like, which ultimately impacted my friendships and my self-esteem.

Finally I was carefree, with only myself to worry about. I wasn't even looking for a partner at this point of my life, as I was focusing on who I wanted to be and enjoying myself.

I was at a good friend's house one afternoon, having afternoon tea. This friend I've known since I was at school, and she has been in the same relationship since her late teens. She was married in her early twenties to a lovely man, and they had their family home set up, with their first young daughter only two years old. She had experienced some trouble conceiving originally, so she already understood the challenges that many face when trying to start a family. Me, I was still oblivious to all of this, and had not thought further of starting a family at this point. In fact it was not a priority at all at this stage in my life.

My good friend asked me about my life; did I have a boyfriend, why not, am I putting myself out there? All those fabulous yet imposing questions you love to hear from a happily married person when you're single. I was nonchalant in my responses, and tried to change the subject. Then the real killer question came, the one that stuck with me for a while.

'Have you thought about freezing your eggs?' She asked me in a way that was light and airy, yet I saw the intent in her eyes. I remember looking at her confused, not really sure where she was going with this. I kind of laughed, brushing it off as a joke. But she was serious.

'You know you're thirty now, and your chances of conceiving decrease year after year. Even if you met someone now, you might not be married for a couple of years. You should think about freezing your eggs. You don't want to lose your chances of having a baby in the future'. She was so direct, something I loved about this friend, and sometimes she was right to be.

That conversation still replays in my head, and to be honest I cannot remember what I said in response. It wasn't something I had ever thought of, and I didn't see it as something I should be worried about at thirty. Would you?

Anyway of course I didn't take the advice. It didn't even start me in a mad panic to find my future husband. I carried on with my lifestyle, moving again interstate within a few months for my next career opportunity, and in my early thirties I moved again, this time overseas to further pursue my career and my personal ambitions, to travel and find adventure.

Well, I'm happy to say that all my eggs stayed firmly in my ovaries, waiting for the day that I would finally settle down, opting for the natural way of starting a family. Perhaps it was the 'au naturel' way to approach my family options, but I was comfortable with that at the time, and I still am now.

Tick-Tock-Tick-Tock.

One final incident that stays with me happened after I had met my now husband. We were both around mid-thirties, and had been together just over a year having just moved in together. We were enjoying our life as a 'young' couple with financial freedom. We enjoyed champagne dinners out, romantic weekends away, travelling to new and exotic destinations and just enjoying life with no real responsibilities. We were also saving for our first home together.

We were out for dinner one evening at a small local restaurant. Another couple were at the table beside us, and somehow during the meal we started conversing with them. I'm not really sure how it happened, but I ended up in conversation with just the woman, as my husband and her partner engrossed themselves in their own banter about cars. She had been telling me that they had been married now for several years, she was over forty and that they were desperate to start a family. Due to her age, she was seeing her chances to conceive a baby start to diminish, having tried several options including a number of rounds of IVF. Nothing had been successful for them so far.

This woman was doing most of the talking. She had indulged in a couple of glasses of wine, and was now sharing personal details about her life with me, many of which she volunteered openly. For me this wasn't the dinner conversation I was expecting. Mostly I nodded and smiled, and just listened. It was when she turned on me with questions about me that I became edgy. 'What's your situation?' I recall just laughing it off, relaying the string of comments that usually came out when these questions were asked; we are happily enjoying our life as a couple, no real commitment yet, we will take it all as it comes. That was it, her face changed, and it was apparent. What I had said was so abhorrently wrong. She turned her chair to place her entire body in front of me, and gripped both my hands to turn my body to face her directly.

'What's stopping you?' she asked me intently. I kind of looked around her nervously; I wasn't sure how I should respond. I tried quickly to gain eye contact from my husband but he was deep in discussion.

'I'm not sure?' I answered tentatively. I really wasn't sure what she wanted me to say. What was the right answer here?

'You need to start trying now or you will regret it.' She was so direct, and absolutely resolute in her convictions.

'Ah… Well, we really aren't ready… We're not married, we want to save, buy a house, we want to travel…' I was rambling, but it was true. It wasn't something we had spoken about. I was looking intently towards my husband hoping he'd pick up on my discomfort, what was being said, and try to distract us and stop this train wreck of a conversation from getting any worse. No hope!

'Why? What's going to change except that your chances of having a baby will become less and less. You need to just start now. I now regret never starting earlier in my life. Now I may never have children. Do you want to be like me?' This woman was starting to scare me a little, and in fact, I realised that anything I did say except, 'Yes of course we'll start trying tonight,' wasn't going to subdue her. It was at this point I started to subtly kick my husband under the table in a 'save me please' way. In the meantime I just continued to smile and nod as she continued to detail her infertility and IVF challenges, whilst telling me that we should just start making babies immediately, that night even! My husband got the message eventually and he intervened, starting a random conversation about dessert choices. The rest of the conversation stayed pleasant and non-topical until the bill arrived.

The sad thing is that this woman had been through years of challenges in trying to conceive, and I really hadn't appreciated at that time in my life how emotionally and physically draining the baby-making process could be. Reflecting back on her reaction and comments, I can understand her desperation, and her best intentions to save me from what she had gone through. My reaction at the time was shock, a little bemusement even. I really hadn't understood why she was so intent that I change my views and my timeline to start a family.

I remember walking home with my husband, sharing with him the story. He had no idea that this conversation was taking place between me and this woman, he had heard nothing. We had laughed about what we felt was her extreme behaviour and brushed it off as a bizarre night. We didn't really talk about having children or marriage at that point. We were happy and that was what mattered for where we were in our relationship at that point in time.

I wonder what would have happened had I taken this woman seriously. Granted we were together and in a stable relationship, and we were committed to each other. Financially we had the ability to start a family, and we were both level-headed, mature individuals. There really weren't any other excuses at this point, except that we were enjoying ourselves, and we had plans to buy a home, potentially get married, and then start a family in that order. Again a choice was made to disregard the comments of an eccentric woman, and carry on with life as normal.

At the same time we had friends starting their families around us at this stage, and we also watched their lives change dramatically as their children took over. We weren't ready at this stage for such an emotional commitment, and that was our choice. I could never regret the choice we made back then, as it wasn't meant to be our time.

Whilst I knew they lived locally, I never had the opportunity to meet that couple again. I will never know if they finally achieved their hope of starting a family. I like to think that they did achieve success, and that they now have their rainbow baby. It's important that I believe there is a reason why we are challenged in life at times, that it's just one hurdle, before great things to come, and that life holds a destiny for all of us.

Best Laid Plans

Ever since I was a young girl, like many young girls, I had dreamed of getting married and having children. I wrote a diary when I was sixteen years old, and I laughed a few years ago as I read through it, reminiscing on my dreams. I was going to be married by twenty years old to a rich European business man, with twin girls at twenty-one. I'd even picked out baby names. OK, so I married an Irishman (I count that as European), but I was thirty-five before I walked down the aisle. Everything seems so easy when you're young, so straightforward, and there is so much to look forward to, so many things to aspire to, it's hard not to get excited about it all, and think that it will all be attainable.

The dream of family and children never really left me though, although the timeline kept creeping back. I always knew it would be something that I would want, to fulfil my life dreams, create my legacy.

Almost two years into my relationship with my now husband, a small hiccup to that plan arose. We had planned an intimate, romantic dinner for Valentine's Day at a local Michelin star restaurant. We'd been living together over eight months now, and as two very independent individuals moving in together we had now just started to feel like a partnership. I'm not really sure how the conversation directed itself this way, but as we were paying the bill we started to discuss our future. We hadn't really talked about it in detail previously, and I guess because I was starting to feel more confident in us together, it was the right time.

So I asked, 'Where do you see us going? As a couple?' Yes I know, that's the question that every man is supposed to dread. I could see his eyes roam the room madly as the words left my mouth. It was out there now, he had nowhere to go; he had to respond.

'I see you in my future, us together for a very long time,' he said and tried to then change the subject. I stayed firm.

'What about marriage? Children?' I continued the cross-examination, but it was better to have the conversation now, in the moment; it was the right time. His answers floored me.

'I've never seen myself getting married, I'm not sure I will, and I don't want children.' He was so matter of fact, so sure. I was dumbfounded. How had I never seen this before? He was from a divorced family, so I knew his view of marriage wasn't positive, but surely he didn't think this was how all couples ended up?

'Well, I want marriage and I definitely want children one day,' I announced firmly. We left the restaurant and started walking back to our house. The conversation continued.

'I'm honestly not sure if I'll want to get married, and if I do it would be at least a few years away,' he explained, 'and I can never see myself being a parent, I don't like kids, and I don't think I'd ever be a great parent. I don't have the patience.'

I didn't respond. In fact, we continued walking in silence as I processed what he had just said. I started to cry. I loved this man with all my heart, but my mind went into turmoil as I considered what my life would be like if I agreed to never get married, never have any children. Marriage aside, I knew I wanted to one day be a mother. Not right then, at that time, but one day. I couldn't imagine agreeing to put those dreams aside, yet I couldn't imagine not being with him.

'I'm sorry I can't change my feelings,' he said as we walked, seeing that I was upset.

'I'm not asking to change you,' I said tearfully, trying to catch my breath, as I was starting to feel that this was all falling apart, we were falling apart. 'I want children no matter what, I want to be a mum one day; it's my dream, I can never imagine that not happening.' I was getting anxious, unsettled, but I needed to say this. We had to have this conversation.

'I'm not sure what I can say. I do love you, but I can't promise you something that I don't want.' That was it; he couldn't give me what I wanted. I also didn't want to wake up in twenty years' time resenting him for not giving me what I wanted. There was no easy way.

'I need to make a choice then,' I said, and I could hear myself sounding a little hysterical. My crying hardened and I just looked around at where we'd been walking. We were a block away from our house; it was past eleven at night but I just needed to get away from this moment. As we turned the corner, I just ran, ran away from him, and away from the conversation. I needed some alone time, and it sounds a bit reckless, a female running away to god knows where at that time of the night, but I needed to be by myself. I heard him call after me but I ignored it, and just ran. I found a small, dimly lit park nearby and a park bench where I sat. I had my mobile with me, and whilst it wouldn't protect me from danger, I felt safer having it with me. It kept buzzing as my partner kept calling, texting. I texted back, a short, brief message, saying, 'I'm OK, be home in thirty minutes, just need to be alone right now.' I didn't want to panic him, but I didn't want to be around him right now.

I realised that I had to be strong here in what I did next. I had a choice. I could stay with him, but I'd have to suffice with never having children, maybe not getting married. If I was to agree to that option under his terms, I couldn't be the woman who regrets it in the future, and I couldn't hold it against him, as my dreams were never going to be realised. Our relationship would never last that.

The only other choice, one that pained my heart as I thought it through, was to leave now, end our relationship. If this man couldn't give me the family I really wanted, and I couldn't let go of that dream, it was better to go now, walk away rather than create a future of hurt and resentment. I cried so hard in that park on my own, feeling as though I would never be strong enough to get through this. I cried myself out, letting all my emotions drain the tears from my eyes. I then picked myself up and walked back to the house.

My partner was in the living room waiting for me as I entered the house. I could see he was also upset. This wasn't easy for him, but he had been truthful and I respected that. I gave him my choice, my reasons for that choice that I couldn't stay in a relationship where we didn't have the same dreams, that I loved him and didn't want us to end up resenting each other because we wanted different things. We spoke, we cried, and he told me to not to make a decision tonight, that he loved me and didn't want to hurt me. I knew that was true above all things.

We went to bed that night with a dark cloud hanging over us, as we couldn't go back to the way things were. Over the next week, I started to think about how I would cope as a single woman again, and what I should start doing if we did leave each other. I'd confessed the story to a good friend, told her that I was thinking of my options as a single woman, and that I would even look at starting a family on my own if I never met 'Mr Right'. She respected that this was the hardest decision of my life, to leave a man I loved dearly, for a dream I had created for my life as a little girl.

As the week progressed, my partner and I spoke in great detail a number of times. It was always very emotional, and I know he was seeking solace and advice from his many friends, both married and single. It was the following weekend when we had a serious talk about making my decision a reality. I didn't want this to drag on, and the longer I stayed the longer I felt that I would give in, and hope he would just change his mind. But I couldn't be certain of that, and this was a decision we both had to make. I told him I would need to leave the house sooner rather than later, as staying there was breaking my heart every day.

'Don't leave,' he said, truly hurting too. I could see it plainly in his face, his eyes. Both of us didn't want this to end this way. We did truly love each other, and we knew that we made a good couple, a strong partnership. It was obvious to me very early on in our relationship that this was the man I wanted to spend the rest of my life with, and I was confident that he felt the same way too.

Over that week, my partner had also spent a lot of time thinking, reflecting on what he wanted in his life, his future with or without me. 'I do want you in my life; I want us to stay together I know that. I love you very much! I see us together for a very long time, buying a house together. I had just never thought of family, and I'm not good with kids in general, so I never thought of me having my own.' He was talking wholeheartedly, without barriers. This wasn't like him to be emotive; I'd normally have to torture him to say anything remotely gushy. 'I have thought about it, and if you want children, I'll do my best to be a good father. I know that when we have our own it will be different, and I want a future with you.' I didn't expect that at all! I also knew he wasn't just saying these things to make the situation go away for now. He was being honest, and he was committing to a future with me, family included.

'I don't want you doing anything you'd regret. I don't want to force you into something you don't want.' I was crying again. I really did love this man, and I wanted this to work with all my heart.

'You're not forcing me. I love you enough to know that if I were to have children, I'd want to have them with you.' He was being earnest, and I knew this was a most important turning point in our relationship. We weren't talking about starting straight away, or getting married tomorrow. It was talk of what could be for our future, a hope that we would one day be a growing family unit.

So as you may have guessed, we didn't break up at that point in time. In fact our relationship grew stronger from that moment on, more honest and more open. We made an offer on our first house later that year, and moved into our new home together in October. It was the December in that same year, just before Christmas, when my partner got down on one knee and asked me to be his wife. I didn't hesitate, my answer was of course a 'most definitely!' We were married just under twelve months later, and it was truly one of the best days of my life. Dreams can come true!

Let's Get This Party Started.

We were married almost a year when we finally decided to 'try' to have a baby. It seemed like the 'right' thing to do, and we were in no hurry. I guess we had assumed this would be a lot easier. Up until then, I was on the pill, and had been for many years. For me, I was going to stop taking the pill one day and voila, baby would appear nine months later... Right? Wrong! I had no idea how this would work, but I had this fantastical notion that it just would.

We left for our dream holiday to the Maldives, and I had left that contraceptive pill packet at home, throwing chance to the wind, believing for sure that we would be pregnant and telling our friends and family the exciting news on return from holiday. Naïve you say? I certainly was!

We naturally had many opportunities on this holiday to make it happen, but not surprisingly my period arrived shortly after we returned from holiday. To be honest, I really didn't know much about the pregnancy journey, and I was thinking that it was potentially several bouts of good sex, and the timing and results would then just magically work themselves out.

I had heard so many stories of women who 'accidently' fall pregnant, so I assumed my own experience would be a piece of cake. However, I quickly realised that more information was needed on how this 'trying to conceive' notion worked. Unbeknown to me this was the world I had avoided for many years, as my intention was always 'not to get pregnant', and at this point in time, I had to do a complete about face, landing smack bang into our new focus – get pregnant quick! I was, after all, thirty-six and to me time was definitely running out!

Whilst it was still all about enjoying the baby-making sex, which of course is the fun part, it was now also about timing, tests, symptoms, positions, and sometimes just watching a calendar month on month, and then waiting for the next cycle. Suddenly there was the realisation that having a baby is pretty serious business, life changing and something we couldn't just be frivolous about. The entire process made me more appreciative of the responsibilities and commitment that beheld parenthood, and what it would really mean to be a parent one day, hopefully.

What Did Google Say Next?

Firstly I'd like to say that the Internet has become such an amazing information tool, and I really don't know how we lived without technology like Google in the past. Nonetheless, it can be a dangerous play toy for someone with limited knowledge, looking for answers, with the time and inclination to search on topics that sit at the front of our mind.

Just try an internet search on 'trying to get pregnant'. It is mind-blowing, the information, articles, blogs, forums, visuals and information that are available. I started on a journey of discovery finding things I never knew had existed, and suddenly entered a world of terms and concepts that are unbeknown to most.

Really! When I started 'trying' I had no idea about what my cycle was, when the best time was to have sex, what signs I should be looking for, or even that there were actually different types of cervical mucus. Yes that's right, there are actual subtle changes you need to monitor as you start to ovulate and it's a process of daily checking.

There were also acronyms I'd never heard of, and through time I started to actually use them in my everyday life.

DTD (Doing The Dance) – that means having sex

TTC (Trying To Conceive) – yep, that's the aim

AF (Aunt Flow) – the strangest name for your period

BFP– what we all want to get, our Big Fat Positive test result

BFN – the opposite of the above, when you get a negative test, and, sigh, start the cycle again!

This is just the tip of the iceberg and I could go on all day. There are actually forums with full reference pages to the acronyms used throughout the conversations. It's like another world, a different language, and soon enough I was actually speaking it too!

The Internet also brings a light on the paranoia, worries, challenges and the emotional rollercoaster many women experience in their efforts to become mothers.

This was suddenly a new world that I was entering, one where previously I hadn't paid attention to my period cycles, or what days were best to conceive, and when should I start testing or symptom spotting.

Looking back at the very start of this phase, I remember getting excited over the silliest signs that I could perhaps be pregnant. Sometimes I knew I was overthinking symptoms, and certainly imagining symptoms that weren't there.

One example that is commonly cited on the Internet as a clear early pregnancy sign is the increased tenderness of your boobs. So having read this, and leading up to my period due date, I must have pinched my nipples so much and so often, that they were starting to bruise blue and purple from the regular squeeze torture I was inflicting on them. Anyone watching me must have thought I was obsessed with touching my own boobs! And of course, because they were constantly being squeezed, they were tender. Most certainly this led me to believe that I must indeed be pregnant.

The truth of the matter was that I was actually killing each and every nerve cell in my poor nipples through my constant pinching and poking, and lo and behold, when that month's test came back negative, I was crushed! Devastated!

And then the next month's cycle would start again, and my obsession would start over with it.

This wasn't the only thing the Internet offered up for hopeful ladies like myself. There's a myriad of forums and discussion groups, where women offer their own 'expert advice', each contradicting the next, and the problem is that as a new expectant mum, with no experience of pregnancy, you believe everything that the Internet tells you. It must be the truth if someone else experiences it.

The discussion forums and groups on the Internet are vast, and you can join a forum if you're trying to conceive, newly pregnant based on your due date, if you've miscarried, or trying after a miscarriage. There are literally forums on every pregnancy and post pregnancy topic available. Every forum has plenty of members, and these members are vocal.

My biggest problem was that at each step of the pregnancy, I would sit on the Internet, Googling answers, like I was going to get that one response with the miracle solution I was looking for. The one response that would make my ultimate dream of being a mother come true.

If things were going wrong, I would feel as though someone else out there in the Internet world had also experienced exactly the same. I had favourite pages set up on my iPad, and before long, it became my right arm. After all, the Internet was always right! That's what I'd convinced myself.

All The Symptoms Say What?

It's funny how unaware I had been about my body, my cycle and what happens throughout, before I started trying to conceive! I truly had believed that I would just do a pregnancy test and, bam, I'd see that double line, that word 'pregnant' flash, and all would be done.

The only symptom I was aware of was morning sickness, but that was par for the course as a part of early pregnancy. However, as I Googled more about pregnancy, I was made aware of so many more potential symptoms that could indicate an early pregnancy.

Now, as you know, for women trying to conceive the cycle is generally twenty-eight days. It is all just a timing and waiting game, right? Waiting for that big 'O', ovulation, to occur. Then at around the two week mark, it's the symptoms that show ovulation: mild cramping; gooey, clear cervical mucus (sorry, way too much information); increase in temperature; and for me an increased sexual appetite.

Then there's the 'two week wait'! Another concept I'd never heard of before, but when you're trying to conceive it's like slow torture, and time dragging its heels. It was like waiting for Christmas Day to arrive as a child, being stranded at the side of the road waiting for the next bus, or the frustration of being wide awake on a long haul flight with a broken entertainment system. I was wishing my days and weeks away, finding it hard to concentrate at work, and just spending my nights on trying to conceive baby forums sharing my impatience with other women in the same position.

All of a sudden I was counting days past ovulation and anticipating my period due date, which was clearly marked on my calendar, and each day teasing me with real or fake symptoms.

The symptoms or 'perceived' symptoms were the worst. So at each day past ovulation, apparently, some sites say that there are signs, and early pregnancy symptoms can start. Well, of course I was positive that I had everyone one of them, and that each symptom was a sure sign that this time I would get my 'big fat positive' test result.

Every month I created my own anxieties and built up the anticipation, awaiting the day my period might be due, wishing and hoping that it wouldn't arrive. I had a handful of common pregnancy symptoms I would monitor and sometimes imagine, and in that way, it would be all consuming, filling my thoughts every moment, all day long. These symptoms were my hope.

1. Fatigue. Now the question was whether this was early pregnancy fatigue, or the fact that I'd stayed up half the night reading forum activity, worked about fifty hours that week, or that I kept waking myself up during the night because suddenly I was sure I needed to pee more frequently.

2. More frequent urination, which of course meant that something was growing inside me, right? Even though at three to four weeks a foetus is less than a millimetre in size, surely something was of course putting more pressure on my bladder. Of course it wasn't the fact that I was drinking water all day long, because I was thirsty.

3. Thirst! So I had heard that thirstiness is a sure sign of early pregnancy. Suddenly my taste buds were changing. I continually refilled my bottle of water at work, and took a large glass of water to bed with me.

4. Breast tenderness. We covered that one in the earlier chapter, and by now the bruising on my nipples had spread, and although I generally get tenderness around my period, this time it definitely felt different.

5. Darker nipples. Well, with all that pinching of course they looked different, more swollen. But then

again, it of course could be a sign that I really was pregnant this month!

6.   Nausea. Every time I ate, or didn't eat, I waited for that feeling, that feeling that maybe my stomach didn't feel settled, or did it? Is that my stomach lurching, what does the nausea feel like?

7.   Cravings and strange tastes. Suddenly I need chocolate mid-afternoon, that's a craving for sure! Now I know I'm pregnant because I didn't need a chocolate last week, and this week it tastes so much better than it has before. It's not because I skipped breakfast this morning, because I thought I felt ill due to nausea. No of course not!

8.   Cramping. So leading up to my period due date, small cramps would start in my lower abdomen. A sure sign of pregnancy in all the books and websites, but then again, could it just be an early sign of my period arriving also? No, definitely not my period.

9.   Late period. Every twenty-eight days my period would generally arrive like clockwork, except when it arrived at twenty-nine days or thirty. But this month, it wasn't there on the morning of day twenty-eight. Excitement! I'm pregnant! Test done and it's negative. Sure enough, that dreaded period would catch me later that day or early the next.

Nonetheless for that moment in time before it arrived, I would be positive this was the month, and the pregnancy test was just slow to respond.

Through each cycle, in those early stages, my hopes would be lifted. I'd convince myself that I was pregnant whilst always creating an internal debate with myself, trying to reason with reality. I would tell myself that I was misreading the symptoms, trying to manage my expectations, but still secretly hoping that this time I was wrong. I would be hoping for that one positive result that would change our lives forever.

Each website, reference book or information sheet has a different list of symptoms, and many of them I haven't referred to. Symptom-spotting became a regular process, always on my mind in each cycle and convincing myself to believe that these were strong signs of a pending pregnancy.

I realise I was lucky; many women spend a good year or so trying before they get their first positive pregnancy test. Regardless of how my pregnancies turned out, I was able to fall pregnant relatively quickly, compared to some women.

After seven months of trying we were very fortunate and excited to finally get a positive pregnancy test result. For me, seven months was a lifetime, and whilst each month I had focused on my cycle and started to understand all of my body patterns, it still took me by surprise.

An unexpected surprise, as the moment you see that positive test it all feels quite surreal, like you never dreamed it actually would or could happen. A lovely surprise, and a moment of excitement, anticipation, hope and joy that I really cannot describe.

It was then, when I finally was pregnant, that those symptoms I was desperately hoping would arrive, actually did. From there, the next hurdle hit, and it's what I call the symptom rollercoaster.

Every pregnancy is different, and with each pregnancy, symptoms can come and go. However, as a newly pregnant woman, that's where the real insecurities and paranoia set in, as you read the ups and downs of every symptom, overthinking positive and negative outcomes. Thinking the worst is the hardest thing not to do, and it then becomes so much harder as the stakes suddenly became higher. If I had thought the symptoms ruled my world whilst trying to conceive, I was completely misled. The pregnancy symptoms after that elusive positive test were now my every waking thought, and a girl could go insane with the battle of internal thoughts and worries in those early stages of pregnancy.

To Test or Not to Test

Achieving that elusive BFP (the positive pregnancy test result) is one step forward. From there everything should really be 'happy days' of planning, excitement and simply just breathing an extra-large sigh of relief. Well, I thought that to start, and then paranoia sank in.

The reality of seeing the result of that pregnancy test was completely overwhelming. I couldn't stop staring at the small test strip, and I couldn't believe my eyes. I remember the first time so clearly. My husband was away with work, and earlier that week I had been sick with food poisoning or some stomach bug. At the time I actually had thought maybe I was pregnant, but I was so ill, I went to the doctor. Before they did any tests, I did warn them that I could be pregnant. The nurse asked me when my period was due. It was a Tuesday, and I said it was due Thursday. So she asked me for a urine sample. She did not seem enthusiastic at all about my potential pregnancy, and I was so put out by her sombre mood. I was holding hope that this was my month, regardless of the fact that my stomach was turning me inside out with pain. Hope was still there!

She took the urine sample away and left me in the waiting room with a glass of water and vomit bowl. I was not well at all. When she returned, her sombre mood arrived again with her.

'Well, you're not pregnant,' she advised me in a matter-of-fact manner. And she handed me some drugs to take, including a painkiller. I was deflated, but took her handful of drugs and swallowed them obligingly. I was sent home a few hours later, feeling a little more in control of my stomach and in less pain.

I rested for the following two days and felt much better for it. But I still didn't feel 'right'. By the Friday I hadn't thought much of my pending period, and I knew sometimes it could be a day or two late. But given that the nurse so bluntly told me I was not pregnant, I really didn't even contemplate the possibility. However that afternoon, driving home after work, the thought suddenly crossed my mind again. Maybe? No it couldn't be, I told myself. After being so ill, how could I be? I was being silly.

Regardless, I did stop by a pharmacy and picked up some vitamins for health, and a pregnancy test. When I got home I chastised myself for being so hopeful, and decided not to test that night, and to wait and see if my period arrived in the morning. I was getting little cramp pains, so it could be arriving any minute now.

My husband was also arriving back late afternoon on the Saturday, so I had a quiet Friday night by the television, and put the entire thing out of my mind. It would be a waste of a perfectly good test, when I was convinced that my period was well on its way.

I woke early the next morning and lay in bed for a bit. I knew my period hadn't arrived, and my own internal debate started to emerge. Should I just test? Was I being silly? Why wouldn't I wait until my husband arrived home? Surely he should be here if it is that amazing moment? We could be excited together. But what if it was negative again? He would just think I was really silly, testing when I had a negative test earlier this week.

Then I just bounded out of bed, went straight to the bathroom and pulled out that test. Something came over me. I had to know, I was torturing myself thinking it could go either way, and really I didn't think it would come up roses for me this time, so I might as well just get it over with. Well I was wrong.

Within moments, the shock hit me as that test came up with a 'Pregnant – 1–2 weeks'!

'Oh my god!' I squealed in disbelief, but no one was around to celebrate. I looked at the time; it was five thirty a.m. Seriously? It couldn't be that early, could it?

What the hell! I thought, I'm calling my husband. His sleepy, grumpy 'hello' answered the phone after several rings. He'd clearly been out the night before, and my phone call had ruined a small sleep in before his flight home!

'We're pregnant!' I said excitedly. I didn't even give him the chance to wake up properly.

'What?' he questioned. I wasn't sure he had fully comprehended my statement. 'How do you know? What?'

'I just did a test, my period was late, the test is positive. Are you excited?' Words were just flying out, but I couldn't contain myself.

'I am excited,' he reassured me, 'great news, how are you feeling?'

'I'm so happy!' I said enthusiastically. 'Can't wait for you to get home!' I was optimistic and my shrill excitement must have sounded a little hysterical through the phone, I didn't care, I was elated, and I wanted my husband to be a part of this thrilling moment.

We ended the call quickly. There wasn't much more to say over a telephone; I think we were both just in a little shock. It had actually happened, at last. We were pregnant! The rest of the day was a blur; I was like a child on Christmas morning. I couldn't sit still and the smile on my face was unmovable; my cheek muscles were aching but I didn't care!

I was on cloud nine all day. Suddenly I started thinking about my due date and other key dates that I needed to start diarising. I started planning the months ahead, and I could see myself thinking about what maternity clothes I would be wearing in what season, what our nursery could look like, and then there were child seats, prams, and other baby essentials. Online shopping here I come! It was all happening for me and my husband, and we would be parents!

I let my hands rub my non-existent bump, as I thought happily about my stomach growing, nice and round. It all seemed quite unreal and I just couldn't wait for the months to pass until I was waddling along, unable to see my toes, with a floaty dress and swollen feet. This was what it was all about, and suddenly it was happening to us. This was our time!

Doctor 'Uh Oh'...

I booked myself straight into my GP for an appointment, three days after that positive pregnancy test result. I was confident that my doctor would be as excited as I was. He was seated at his desk when I walked into his consulting room, and I couldn't hold back.

'I'm here because I'm pregnant,' I said proudly.

'How far are you?' His enthusiasm wasn't showing, and his tone was very serious.

'I'm just over four weeks,' I told him.

'OK, so there is nothing I can do for you right now, and in fact you probably should have waited a few weeks to make this appointment. One in three pregnancies end in miscarriage.'

I just stared at him. I couldn't believe his blunt bedside manner. I honestly did not know how to respond to what he had just said. I hadn't even contemplated miscarriage! I knew people who had miscarried, but surely this wasn't going to happen to me.

'How old are you?' he asked, completely ignoring my shock to his earlier statement.

'Thirty-six?' I said hesitantly.

'Hmm, yes you're in the mature age bracket, so I won't book anything in until you reach six or seven weeks. If you're still pregnant then, we can book you in to see a midwife.'

Still pregnant? I decided at this moment that I hated this doctor! No hesitation. I can't remember the rest of the appointment, or what was said by whom next, I just remember feeling so angry, upset, emotional and overwhelmed. This guy was a complete arse! No congratulations, no reassurance, not even a bloody smile! How on earth did he get into this profession and where was the patient empathy and care?

He clearly felt I had wasted his time with my happy news. I may not have had to go to see him at that point of time, and perhaps I was a little early in making an appointment. But I had no idea what to do! This was my first pregnancy. When I looked on the government health website, it said, 'make an appointment with your GP', so I did just that, I was following instructions.

As I walked away from the GP surgery, I assured myself that I would do anything to avoid appointments with this grumpy sod of a doctor again, and I satisfied myself with the fact that I was pregnant, and happy.

Nothing was going to ruin this exciting moment for me.

Testers Anonymous

The home bought, pharmacy pregnancy test is pure evil genius. The manufacturers are onto a great thing here, especially for the paranoid, overthinking, unsure, and newly pregnant consumer market.

You would think that once you get that positive home test result that would be it. You are pregnant, and the test confirms this. Sit back now, relax and enjoy the next nine months.

Well, after my friendly doctor's visit, my paranoia started to rise a little. I googled 'miscarriage for women at the age of thirty-six and upwards'. I also searched the Internet on the topic of 'miscarriage' in general. I trawled through many of the online forums and the latest feeds and discussions, where other women at my stage of pregnancy were still testing and then getting fainter lines? What? Fainter? Can it just go away? These thoughts started emerging and my fears started rising. Maybe my grumpy doctor had a point? Surely not!

So as I was passing the pharmacy I bought another box with two tests in it. I wanted to see that positive result again, reassure myself that all was good in my pregnancy. That's not too strange is it?

I went home and peed on that stick. The apprehension of that first test returned as I waited that three long minutes again, and suddenly the thought hit my head. What if this one came back negative?

Well, of course it didn't. The test quickly flashed 'Pregnant', and this time it said '2–3', meaning my pregnancy was progressing. Yes! I knew it, I was being ridiculous. But still I was very pleased that I had decided to test. It relaxed me, quelling the myriad of thoughts that had been running through my head.

Funnily enough however, that delirium didn't stay. I still had one test left in that pack I bought, and several days later, when my symptoms were going up and down, I pulled out that remaining test stick and peed on it again. I wanted to reassure myself, and I wanted the excitement of watching the word 'Pregnant' appear again. I wasn't disappointed, this time it appeared really quickly, which made me even happier.

By the way, of course it does: as your pregnancy progresses your HCG levels also increase, making the test validate the pregnancy quickly. This should happen, but it was the little things like this that helped me through the nervous points. Also this time, the test progressed even further, and I got the all exciting '3+' result! I breathed a sigh of relief, took a photo of the test with my iPhone as a keepsake, and sent it to my husband in a text message.

His response by text? '*xx*'.

Hmmpphh! No enthusiasm whatsoever. He had no idea of the inner turmoil that had been going through my mind until then. I did appreciate that my husband was incredibly excited about the pregnancy, but his view was that I was completely mad for spending more money on tests when we knew we were pregnant. The first test had a positive result, and he could not understand why I would want to continue doing more tests. It didn't make sense to him, and I was sure it was just a male thing!

The testing addiction happened throughout all my pregnancies. You would think I would have learned my lesson, but alas, the addiction got worse each time. I tested, and retested, loving to see that positive line appear and appear again. And I would obsess that if I didn't test I may just not be pregnant. I'm sure that there is some support group out there for people like me?

During my other pregnancies I would watch the line slowly get darker each time on the first response tests. I would even line them up by day on a piece of paper to showcase my growing pregnancy. I would also buy the more expensive digital tests and strategically time my testing so that I could watch it progress week by week until eventually I received the '3+' on that little display screen, making my heart flip a little and confirming that everything was actually progressing. That for me was the focus of my actions and nothing could deter me! It was an addiction, and I must have spent a small fortune on different test products, but I didn't care.

My husband, my family and my friends all thought I was absolutely crazy, but I couldn't be told. I even tested the progress of my pregnancies in secret, hiding the results, so that my loved ones couldn't comment on my crazy addiction. I guess it was the one thing that maintained my reassurance in those early weeks, and it was my way of coping.

Patience is a Virtue

I had set up an application on my phone, a pregnancy tracker. It gave me daily updates on my pregnancy, how big baby was from the size of a grain at five weeks, developing into a grape by seven weeks. It gave me hints and tips on food and exercise, and every morning I excitedly opened the application to watch my pregnancy progress by day.

It was only March, and I had many months to go, yet this app must have been opened several times a day in anticipation of our baby due in October.

Every day, I turned side on in the mirror and scrutinised my stomach for this bump that would appear hopefully in the coming weeks. I even took a picture of myself side on, thinking I could take one each month and watch myself progress.

I was sure my boobs were getting bigger, and started planning my next bra purchase in the bigger cup size. Something firm but supportive, and I couldn't wait to start thinking about maternity jeans and trousers to allow for a growing bump.

I was at work one day on a conference call that was sending me to sleep, so I started thinking about budgets and planning for purchasing a wide range of 'must have' items for our nursery. I started to create a spreadsheet, and listed the key items we needed to have before our baby would be born. I then reviewed a range of online baby stores for the estimated cost of everything, and created a budget against our savings plan, sending it to the husband for review and approval.

I'm sure that this confirmed to him that I had gone insane as we hadn't even reached the end of our first trimester. Still, I was sure that planning ahead was important, and time felt like it was going so slow at this stage.

We had told a select few friends and family, but I was bursting to tell the world. It felt like a secret I didn't want to keep, as I wanted everyone to be as excited as I was. I couldn't wait until our thirteen week scan, when I could announce our news to friends and work colleagues and of course write a creative post on my social media page.

Each month we had been trying, I watched with anticipation as friends near and far announced their exciting news on their social media pages. Scan photos were posted as profile pictures, and birth announcements with the photos of new born babies only hours old, in their mum or their dad's happy arms were posted, enticing a myriad of congratulatory comments.

That would be us, and I could not wait to share our news and plans openly and proudly. The excitement was literally bursting me at the seams.

It was the day I reached seven weeks and three days, that I understood the reason for the hush and secrecy in the first trimester. I was at work and I went to the bathroom, to find a small amount of blood on my underwear. Emotions overwhelmed me as I suddenly envisioned the absolute worst. I called my husband, who was travelling for work, in a panic, and of course he felt helpless. We agreed I'd make a doctor's appointment.

I was crying in my office when my manager walked by, and of course I had to tell her why I was so upset. She packed me off to the doctor and gave me a big hug of support, wishing me the best and hoping it was just a false alarm. It reassured me that work, regardless of anything else, would be there for me no matter what happened. At this point, I had no idea what to expect next, but I was still hopeful that all would right itself.

It was strange that the feelings of delirium and anticipation could fall away so quickly to helplessness and uncertainty. This was what I found, the regular emotive rollercoaster of pregnancy, which I soon became accustomed to during this pregnancy and others.

A Beating Heart

The doctor's appointment was brief but efficient. She was supportive and understanding and agreed to set me up with an early scan appointment to hopefully provide reassurance that nothing was wrong. The earliest I could get into the early scan unit was the next morning, so I had a twenty-four hour wait in anticipation. I decided that I should not worry and that I could not control the outcome. I was no longer bleeding so that was possibly a good sign.

The next morning I arrived at my local hospital's early pregnancy unit for the scan. Waiting with me were several other expectant mothers, some with their partners. My husband was still away for work, but I was actually OK doing this on my own. I knew he would have been here if he could, and I preferred to get the scan done with rather than wait.

As they called my name, my heart jumped a bit. I was taken into a little dark room with an ultrasound machine, and advised that this would be an internal scan as I was only just past seven weeks. They prepared the table and I prepared myself. A big long dildo type scan object was placed in front of me. That was what they would scan with? The object looked a little intrusive and scary, but I was more scared about what would be seen on the screen.

The sonographer inserted the scan dildo, and I watched her as she intently watched the screen, moving the object from left to right inside me. She seemed to move it into one particular spot and just shifted it slightly around. She would stop and click a button, her expression staying the same. I waited for her to say something, anything. Nothing; this was torture!

The sonographer then asked the second sonographer in the room to come over, and she looked at the screen, shifted the scan dildo a little inside me, and clicked a few more buttons. I watched both of their expressions and I struggled to spot any signals telling me if this would be a good or bad result.

As I lay there, no clothes on my lower half, a foreign object inside me wiggling about, and these two sonographers staring intently at a screen that was out of my view, I thought about the many women who must enter this room, worried and scared like I was today. Where was the patient empathy and bedside manner? Don't get me wrong, I want them to concentrate and take the time to do what they are trained to do, but surely a smile, a couple of words to calm my nerves or just some understanding of what I might be feeling right now wasn't too much to ask?

One of the sonographers finally looked at me and asked me to get dressed. I waited for her to say something else, but she removed the scan dildo, gave me some tissue paper and went to the small desk in the corner of the room. I just nodded, not really sure what to expect, but my gut feeling said that this wasn't good.

Once dressed, I announced that I was ready and asked tentatively, 'What did you see?'

The nurse pulled out a chair beside her, and I sat.

'There is a pregnancy,' she stated, 'it's dating at six weeks and four days, so a week earlier than the dates you've given me.' I nodded, that was still good surely? I tried to keep my hopes up, but her matter-of-fact tone still had me worried.

'However, the heart beat is slow,' she said, again in her monotone voice. 'We will set up a follow up scan for a week, and see if the pregnancy is still viable.'

'How slow?' I asked.

'Slow enough for us to be concerned.' She paused, and could see I needed more detail. 'It may speed up, or it may slow down or even stop; we will know by next week.'

It had a heartbeat, I thought, but what does 'slow' mean at this point of my pregnancy, and it's not as big as it should be? They gave me the scan picture, but it was just a picture of a small blob in a sac. I didn't know how I felt. I called my husband immediately as I knew he'd be waiting for my call. He was reassuring and said we should just wait and hope for the best over the next week.

The next week was tough and the days dragged. I wanted to put the next scan out of my mind, but I was anxious to get the next results, and hopefully move forward with my pregnancy. To my own surprise I was able to remain generally positive that this would work out for us.

I did, however, spend a solid amount of time on Google, looking up, 'slow heartbeat success stories' or 'six weeks and slow heartbeat'. There were sad stories and there were some good news stories. Some of the stories I read said that the foetus was so small at six to seven weeks, and that some ladies had seen a slow heartbeat, returning a week later to see it quicken and beat so loud and so fast, with baby growing. I was hopeful that this would also be the same for us. I still felt pregnant so surely that was a good sign?

I continually reminded myself that I had to remain positive until the next scan and that my little bub was just a slow grower, or maybe I had my dates wrong. Negative thoughts would not help my situation, and my husband was of the same opinion. We now just had to wait and hope, and that week felt like a year as each day dragged its heels to a close.

Nothing Can Prepare

On the day of the second scan, a week later, my husband and I returned to the sonographer's office together. We were hopeful and talking positively about our pregnancy plans. I still felt pregnant with signs of nausea and tender boobs, so I was focused on remaining positive.

We were due to leave for a holiday that weekend with another couple who were also pregnant (about eight weeks in front of us) and we were excited about sharing our news with them. I had thought about how we would compare our pregnancies and have our children grow up together as friends. I wanted to take a picture scan away with us from the appointment today, so that I could show off my little bean to my closest friends and family. I had thought eight weeks was early, but we would want to share the news with our nearest and dearest.

We entered the dark room together and I prepared myself again for the internal scan. As the process started I waited with anticipation, holding my husband's hand tightly as he stood beside me.

The sonographer's face said it all; she didn't have to say the words, and I could see that it was bad news with one look.

'I'm so sorry!' she said. My eyes filled with tears and I felt my heart break with those words.

I breathed in and out, feeling as though the dark walls of the room were closing me in. I felt my husband's hand tighten in my grasp.

'There is no heartbeat, the pregnancy is no longer viable,' she explained sombrely. I couldn't speak; I looked up at my husband who was looking back at me. His eyes were shiny whilst mine watered up as I started to cry. My husband leant down and kissed me.

'When you're ready, you can get up and change and we can talk through the next steps.' The sonographer was sympathetic in her statement but I knew that she must do this a lot. I felt for her; this wasn't a nice job.

It was like the wind had been taken out of me, and everything I was hopeful and excited about had immediately disappeared from our future. We had hoped, prayed, and longed for this pregnancy, and we almost had it. It was there in me growing for at least six weeks. And then it wasn't. All the excitement that came with that exciting moment in time was suddenly taken away, gone.

It was an early pregnancy loss, what they call a 'missed miscarriage' as there were no signals, no real bleeding or pain. The heart just stopped beating and the foetus stopped growing; a miscarriage would result eventually, but the scan had detected this before my body.

For me, nothing felt different, nothing had changed yet. I knew that there had been a small, minute foetus growing inside me, and for a time there had been hope. A dream of a future family was suddenly taken away, ripped from under me and put on a shelf for a future space in time.

It was explained to me as I sat by the sonographer's desk that I had three options. I could wait for the miscarriage to happen naturally, I could take a tablet that would start the miscarriage faster, or I could opt for surgical removal of the pregnancy. She handed me several pamphlets explaining the miscarriage, my options and what I might be feeling right now. I just held them as she walked my husband and I to a small room. She told me a doctor would come and speak to me and we could discuss our options.

We sat in that room and waited. This wasn't a dream, it was real and we were no longer having a baby. We had to make a decision on how I wanted to now lose our baby, empty my womb, and go back to the way things were before I was pregnant, before we were excited and hopeful. But things couldn't just go back, could they? It would be different now, surely. I knew what being pregnant felt like, how could I go back to not feeling pregnant again? It was still there inside me now, but it was gone. My inner thoughts were in turmoil as I sat just staring at the pamphlets and information sheets in my hand. The words were blurry, but I understood I needed to decide.

Our holiday was in five days time, we were flying up north to Scotland – did I want to be experiencing a miscarriage on that holiday? The couple we were going with, did they really want their holiday overrun by a hormonal woman who was dealing with both an emotional and physical loss? I didn't know what a miscarriage felt like, I didn't know what to expect. Would it be really painful? How much blood would I actually lose? The answer seemed clear to me, as my tears fell onto the sheets of paper, blurring the words even more so.

'I'd like to have this surgically removed,' I whispered to my husband. 'I'd like to do it as soon as possible, if possible, and I would still like us to go to Scotland'.

'Whatever you need,' my husband said reassuringly, still holding my hand. I could see he felt helpless, hurt, lost, I was sure that he was struggling also to deal with this, or with what to expect from me. I knew he would be there for me throughout this, and whilst he would not physically understand, he was grieving an emotional loss, a pregnancy that was part of him, but never would be. It was something neither of us had been prepared for.

It was at least two hours before the doctor came in to see us. We had been sat in that small, closed room for two hours on our own, taking in what we had just been told, and we just waited. Unfortunately, the public health system was under-resourced and this was not an emergency situation, but all the same it was a sterile, uncomfortable environment in the best of circumstances.

We went through the motions, the explanation again of what was happening, blood tests, blood pressure, and finally agreement that we would take option three, the surgical removal. To be really honest, I just wanted to leave now, go home, get out of the hospital, and away from this situation.

The main hospital had no surgical places this week, and again this wasn't an emergency, as I guess they felt if it started naturally it saved them a bed for more serious patients. I appreciated that. Nonetheless, I wanted this done as quickly as possible, and I wanted to go on holiday with a new beginning. I wanted to start over again, and try again. This was, after all, a first pregnancy and I knew that there had to be more chances. I was not giving up. It was this mindset that kept me sane, whilst the hospital nurses and doctors took another hour to look at alternative options for the surgical procedure.

A smaller local facility, which specialises in non-emergency day surgical procedures, was available the next day, and I was scheduled in as their last patient. A way forward! I needed to keep focused on what was happening next, rather than what was happening now, and this suited me well.

Big Girls Do Cry

The women who have unfortunately experienced early miscarriage will appreciate that how you deal with the loss is sometimes a little strange to describe.

There were just moments where I lost it completely, and those moments could and did arise sometimes when I least expected it.

The night before our surgical procedure, I was lying in bed by eight p.m. just thinking, dwelling on what could have been and what was no more. I was sad, and tears kept springing to my eyes as random thoughts of plans we had discussed kept bouncing around in my head. But that's to be expected, right?

I lay in the bed rubbing my belly, knowing that what was in there was no longer alive, had stopped growing a week or so ago, and would be removed 'surgically' tomorrow. It sounded so clinical. At the hospital earlier they had given me options, what we wanted to do with the 'pregnancy' when it was removed. There was an option for a burial, but at six weeks, when it was barely a tadpole-like shape, that didn't feel right. They also said they could just destroy it, medically of course, and that just felt so cold, so insensitive. The other option was to cremate the remains along with other anonymous foetuses, other lost babies, although there would be no ceremony. For me, that was just right, and at least it felt as though our lost baby would be given a moment and a process alongside other lost babies. The thought of it brought me to tears, and I just buried my head into my pillow, hoping I would sleep through the night and get through the next day.

My husband was so sweet that evening. I didn't want to leave my bed and I didn't want to move. He brought me dinner in bed and he sat beside me with his own plate of food. We ate and watched the television in mostly in silence. We held each other after dinner, and he put on a movie. I couldn't really concentrate much on the movie, and in fact I was just grateful to let my mind wander a little. We would be OK, I knew it, and we were OK now; it was just sad and a shame, as we were both fit and healthy, and we were ready for this. Another time, I thought, we have many more opportunities, and I was thirty-six, my body didn't know what had hit it after thirty-six years and being suddenly pregnant. Next time would be our time. That helped me fall asleep.

We had an early start the next morning. I had been in surgery before, so I knew what to expect when we'd arrive, and I was just eager now to have this done and move forward.

I was shocked and upset when we arrived at this small local hospital reception; they took my details and directed my husband to a waiting area, showing me the way through to my hospital bed. The waiting room was so sterile, with small chairs and a tiny television showing the morning show. I was being taken towards a long corridor, and I didn't know where it led. I stopped.

'Can my husband not come with me?' I asked the attending nurse.

'No. We don't allow visitors; he can wait or go home and pick you up.' She was so matter of fact, and I just stared at her and then my husband. My eyes just filled with water and I started crying.

'But I want my husband with me.' I knew I sounded like a five year old, but it was true. I didn't know what I was going into, and I didn't want to do this alone.

'I'm here, I'll be here, I'm not going anywhere,' my husband said. Always the peacemaker, he didn't want a fuss, and he wanted me to be OK. He looked helpless, but he was trying to help both the nurse and me in this situation. I'm sure he could see I was on the verge of losing it, but he also could see – which I could not – that this was their standard hospital procedure; this nurse was only doing her job. 'I'll stay here until you're ready, I'm not going anywhere!' he said, reassuring me, holding my shoulders, looking straight into my eyes. He was such strength, and I just cried and nodded. I wasn't happy, but what could I do?

This nurse led me away from my husband into a large open plan area, where there were beds separated by curtains; I was given the one on the end. She was sympathetic but procedural; she gave me the instructions she had most likely given to many a woman that morning and the mornings before. There was a hospital gown I needed to change into, and then I just needed to wait. There was a big white board in view before they pulled my curtains. I could see my surname on the list; I was number seven, the last one. I knew it would be a long wait for my turn, and it was.

As I sat on the bed, I texted my husband periodically with updates, watching and waiting as each woman in this open plan ward was wheeled away into theatre. I heard the nurses gossiping about their weekend, and I kept forcing myself to think forward, of the future, of our next hope. I also cried on my own, because it was easy to do with the curtains pulled and no one there to say or do anything. I cried for what I was about to lose completely, and for what I wasn't sure would happen next.

It was three hours on, and I was still sitting on the hard hospital bed, curtained off to the rest of the ward, waiting. I'd had enough. I called for the ward nurse, and waited. It was a male nurse who arrived to my distressed state. I knew I was probably acting like a child, but I wanted the company of my husband whilst I waited, and to be honest I didn't know how much longer this process would take. He sympathised and before long he was ushering me out to that sterile waiting room, in a hospital dressing gown, so that I could at least sit beside my husband and wait for my name to be called.

I was grateful for this small gesture, as to me it was just sitting there, watching *Jeremy Kyle* or any other daytime rubbish television that helped keep me sane at this point. And then the nurse came back to call my name. It was my turn. My husband squeezed my hand tightly, kissed my cheek and said, 'See you soon, I love you.' His simple words gave me strength to get up and follow the nurse back down the corridor.

It felt like it all happened quickly and I woke drowsy after the procedure, my stomach aching slightly. I had a little bit of bleeding, but other than that, it was done and I felt ready to leave. I wanted to leave.

I was tired from the sedation and I slept that night very well. I had the next two days off work, and I just rested, recovered, always strangely feeling as though the pregnancy had been a dream, as it no longer felt as though any of it had really happened. I looked forward to our holidays as something that would take us away from it all, and I started to focus on a new beginning. I hoped we could try again, praying for a better outcome next time. Moving forward, staying positive was the only way to keep us from the sadness and grieving. We would always remember our first pregnancy, but life moves on, right? In my mind, many women experience miscarriages, and I had known quite a few. This one wasn't for us, but the next one, I had high hopes for.

Searching for Rainbows after the Storm

There were times after the miscarriage where I had felt isolated with my pain and loss. I knew my husband was feeling pain too, and I was always conscious of his feelings, but there were also moments where I felt very alone. I felt that my own body had let us both down, that I had somehow done something wrong along the way or that there was something wrong with me in the first place. At times I wanted to scream out in pain and I wanted to feel and touch what I had lost. Alas, it was a strange place as I did not know our baby. It wasn't even a baby; it was a foetus, and now it was gone, and I had nothing to show for it.

In these moments I always reverted back to the Internet; I frequented the many baby forums available to someone seeking solace. I found a myriad of pages and groups dedicated to those who have miscarried, and it was comforting to connect with people in similar situations whilst not actually disclosing my identity. These forums were filled with women like myself who were also mourning the loss of what could have been, hoping for the next successful pregnancy. These unknown, anonymous women suddenly became a consolation for me – a connection to help me build myself up, get through this dark storm and find a way forward.

Suddenly a new world opened up, the world of those who had tried and lost, those who were trying multiple times, and the strong, brave and resilient women who kept going. They all had one objective that was most dear in their lives: holding their very own 'Rainbow Baby'!

The 'Rainbow Baby' was a new and thoughtful term I was now enlightened to, something that provided hope. It's the baby after the storm, the baby after the pain and loss, it's the healthy, bouncy baby for those couples who have miscarried or lost through pregnancy. On these forums and through many a conversation on topics of post-loss experiences I remained in awe. These women drove hope, faith and encouragement to each other, always focusing on each other's successes and each and every one dedicated and unrelenting towards their ambitions of one day meeting their very own Rainbow Baby.

As I scrolled through the different conversational topics I realised just how naïve I had been about my own situation and my assumption that getting pregnant or starting family would be so easy. So many women have experienced miscarriage and it was eye-opening how common early pregnancy loss actually was. As I started talking to people I knew – friends, family and colleagues – about what had happened I was also astounded at how many had experienced the same or knew of people who had. This seemed to me a well-kept secret, perhaps something not to share openly, but suddenly my eyes were opening to a different world of conceiving, one surrounded by sadness, loss and misfortune.

At my age, having never tried before, and with the odds against me with my history I really should not have been surprised that the first pregnancy did not succeed. In fact, most people said to me that a miscarriage would have been expected given the circumstances. Perhaps I was lucky it happened in these early stages and that it didn't progress past the first trimester. Whilst this didn't make me feel better, it gave me further hope that next time would be more successful. I reconciled that it was my body's way of dealing with the shock of kick starting it into action with the creation of a little human being. After thirty-six years of stagnancy it needed a small practice run perhaps, and next time would be different. Next time we would have our Rainbow Baby!

Standing in the Rain

With the events of the past week and a holiday forthcoming, I felt as though I was being hit with a mixed bag of emotions. Holidays for me are an event, they have always been something I look forward to, plan and revel in. After what had happened, we certainly needed time out away from it all, time to relax and recover, but given what had happened, this didn't feel like a true holiday. It was as though a dark cloud was hanging over us ready to rain, when we should be looking forward to spending time in a place we'd never been before, enjoying lots of sightseeing, fun and laughter with our good friends.

At the same time, I couldn't cancel it. I couldn't face going back to work, I needed time away. I also didn't feel as though I could take 'sick leave' as two days after surgery I was tired and sore, but in my own view I didn't feel that would qualify for a week off work. Perhaps that was just me being the martyr, I'm sure many people do take the time off, time to grieve at least. They are the sensible ones! Hence, this annual leave break actually made good timing given our circumstances, and knowing that our friends would be there to support us, and hopefully take our mind off what had happened, was a good thing.

My body ached from the surgery, and I was experiencing some general ongoing physical issues as a result. I was advised that I should expect to feel tired, a little sore for around a week or two and I had some medication to help with pain and bleeding. These physical impediments did impact a little on our holiday activities, but luckily we were staying in a lovely rural setting, where I could take slow walks and take long drives without too much effort. Most importantly there was time to rest and recover, spending valuable time away with my husband and our two close friends. It was nice. We had some laughs, relaxed by an open fire at night, enjoyed the scenery in long drives during the day, and in effect, it helped us to start moving on.

There were times where my emotions did run high, and I had some moments of good where I'd just forget, thankfully just getting lost in the good moments. I'd forget at that moment that I had been pregnant, and the loss we'd just experienced, and everything for that split-second would feel normal, like it never really happened. Then suddenly, like a trigger, my thoughts would go backwards, the hurt of the loss would hit me, and I'd just feel miserable all over again. It didn't get easier but with each day, I felt I coped a little better with my feelings, which I guess is all part of that healing process.

I won't lie either; being with our friends on holiday, a couple who were expecting, and who were at the time over thirteen weeks into their own pregnancy, was difficult at times. Sometimes I would see her rub her growing belly, or get lost in the conversations they had about their baby plans, and it would make me feel a little sorry for myself as I wished for the same, but I knew it just wasn't our time this time. They were aware and sensitive to our situation, and my friend understood the pain of miscarriage having experienced loss in her two previous pregnancies.

We spoke about what I had gone through, what I felt, and she encouraged me to keep looking forward. My friend did look forward, and what gave me inspiration was that after her losses she was still incredibly positive and now she was carrying the hope of a new born baby. It reminded me that I could also be that lucky in the future, and I needed to carry hope.

I'm sure there were also moments where our friends felt uncomfortable being on holiday with someone who'd suffered loss only a week before, and I probably showed signs of madness at times with my emotions. But good friends are there through the thick and thin, the good and the bad times. It helped having another couple there with us to take our mind off the reality at times. Being part of a small group, in a small cottage in a rural location, I had to engage in conversation and banter; I couldn't just sulk and dwell in my own sadness.

After a week on holiday, relaxing and sightseeing, I was much more positive. There were moments, mostly at night, when I lay there and my mind would allow those thoughts and dreams of what could have been to enter. I had to allow those dreams and thoughts to enter, and then re-focus them on what could be in the future.

You should understand that I am a detailed planner; I like to have a project, a focus, and something I can work or aim towards. I like timelines, objectives, and an agenda. That is how I am in life, in work, in everything. Even when planning our wedding, I was so organised that on the day everything worked like clockwork with me being the calm and relaxed bride. I knew it would be like this for our wedding, as it was a process that required steps, and I could control each of those steps to deliver what they needed to on the day. With pregnancy I was suddenly realising that things were very different. It wasn't black and white; I couldn't put it in a spreadsheet and keep it under control with dates and deliverables.

I therefore had to accept that this was something I wasn't able to engineer to perfection, and my body and my age were not a spreadsheet. I couldn't systematically plan what would happen next, I just had to accept that things would and could happen, and I would then have to deal with them accordingly. That was how I had to cope with this.

Returning to work after my week's holiday was difficult. I hadn't thought it would be, and hadn't really thought much at all about how I would react. Driving into work that morning, my heart lurched, and suddenly as I was closer to the office, I started to tear up again with no warning. I didn't really understand my reaction at first, and when I entered the office and turned on my computer, I found it hard to concentrate. I thought I had turned a corner but today I felt I was reverting. I sat there staring at my inbox, just thinking I could not start anything. I must have sat there for about ten minutes when the sound of a text message broke me out of my trance.

It was my sister-in-law, sending me a good luck message for the day. It read, '*Thinking of you today on your first day back, hope you're ok xx*'. A simple message but thoughtful, and it took me by surprise on a number of levels. My sister-in-law was like a true sister. She had unfortunately also dealt with miscarriage, and so I knew she understood exactly how I was feeling at that moment. She had also understood that the last time I'd sat in this office I was pregnant and hopeful. Today that was gone. When it all came together I was grateful for her thoughtfulness, and I was also lost, as this was when things went back to the way they were before, officially. No more planning, looking at maternity leave dates and getting excited at the prospect of handing over my position as I plan for maternity leave, thinking about how to tell my colleagues, and starting to back pedal on my work ambitions and focus on family. I was back to scratch, starting again.

That first day back at work was strange, difficult, and sombre. Before long however, things did go back to normal, and whilst it was always in the back of my mind, it also remained a hope for us that we would experience pregnancy again. After all, we did fall pregnant in the first place, so something does work, and that was the first step. Next step was to stay pregnant and I remained ever hopeful!

Short Lived but Loved

Our second pregnancy came as a surprise. It was around six months after my first unsuccessful pregnancy and we had been trying ever since. We were away for the weekend, and my period was not due until the Monday. It was the Saturday before my period due date when I had that familiar strange feeling, something was different, and it occurred to me that again, I could be pregnant.

I shelved that feeling for the day, believing that I was overthinking the situation, and that it was all in my head. But that night after a lovely day of sightseeing, a long lunch and a drive through the Irish countryside, that feeling hadn't subsided. As I tried to sleep, the thought kept circling in my head. What if I am pregnant again? I mentally calculated in my head that this could be an April baby. I resolved that if I still felt the same in the morning, I'd tell my husband and we would pick up a pregnancy test.

Well, that Sunday morning, those pulling, tight feelings were still there, and I was positive that this was a pregnancy. It had to be, this would be our time, I thought excitedly! I braved it and calmly hinted at what I had suspected over breakfast to my husband. He immediately suggested we do a pregnancy test, and to my delight he wanted us to purchase a test that day to find out for sure. Now the problem we faced in Northern Ireland was that no shops were open first thing on a Sunday morning.

In fact, we went to several large shopping centres, all of which were not open until after lunch. This was crazy! We were both eager to test now, and we were being forced to wait.

Well, it was a long morning, most of it spent watching the time slowly tick by. We had breakfast, went for a drive, enjoyed some sunshine and stopped for lunch, but all the time my mind kept reverting back to the 'what if I am?'

We finished lunch just after one p.m., and immediately drove to a large supermarket with a pharmacy. Of course I picked up the digital tests, the most expensive; I wanted to know and was not taking the chance on some cheap test. We drove back to where we were staying and I peed on that stick. My husband waited outside the bathroom.

The test flashed for about five minutes, and my eyes glazed as I stared at the little screen, waiting for the result to appear. It then flickered a little, and the result I was waiting for appeared: 'Pregnant'! Before it even had time to show weeks, I ran out of the bathroom to show my husband. We hugged each other, and this time we felt for sure it was the real thing!

We travelled back home later that evening, and that evening I dreamed of a pregnancy that would be successful, my belly growing large and round, and plans for our nursery.

The next morning, a Monday, I was at work and, whilst I still felt pregnant (similar to the feeling I had on Saturday), there was also a nagging feeling that something wasn't right. Probably my paranoia, but it was there. I had no other symptoms, and a 'gut feeling' that something wasn't right. It didn't feel like the same pregnancy I had before. After work, that evening, I decided to test again, with a box of pregnancy test kits I had bought from an Internet site. Somehow I knew that retesting was the best way to reassure my fears, to confirm everything was really OK.

The line on the test was faint, so faint it took a long time to appear, and it was basically transparent. The worry then started to hit. My stomach lurched as I started to fear the worst. I called my GP office first thing in the morning, and made an appointment with the female doctor in surgery. She heard out my fears, and reassured me that it was early. But given my miscarriage earlier this year, she referred me for blood tests that day. I was pleased to know that my fears were being investigated.

My test results came in that evening and the doctor who called from the hospital didn't sound positive. She gave me a HCG figure and said it was low, advising me that I would need to come back for a second test in forty-eight hours, to see if the results doubled. I was advised that if it doubles, the pregnancy is progressing.

Of course, I also tested the next morning with my own tests, and the worrying thing was that the line was even fainter. I was losing hope that this pregnancy was going to last. My husband was, of course, supportive and reassured me that it would be fine, but I could tell he was worried too.

The following morning I went back into the hospital for the second round of blood tests. They said they would call me as soon as the tests came through. I waited all day for the call. By five p.m. I called the hospital seeking answers. I was so nervous, and whilst I knew it was ending, I still had some hope. No one could help me, but they assured me they would call that evening.

I waited through the next few hours; I couldn't eat, think or concentrate on anything! I had fits of tears as I prepared myself to hear the worst, and became more and more frustrated as I waited for that call. At eight p.m. I called the hospital again and they assured me someone would phone back that evening. I stressed to them that I was waiting by the phone, and really wanted someone to call me that evening.

It was nine thirty p.m. when the doctor finally called, and I answered the call on the first ring. I had been clutching my mobile phone so tightly all night, watching it and waiting, and the stress made me feel so tight in the chest. I was hopeful but realistic, and that phone call was the catalyst for our future. Unfortunately the results were lower, significantly so! The doctor on the phone confirmed that the pregnancy was no longer viable, and I would miscarry in the imminent future. The results had dropped below half of what they had been; I was losing this baby too. Another miscarriage, I thought, and everything just went numb again.

He was right. The miscarriage started on its own over the following weekend, two days after I had the results over the phone. I was lucky, the miscarriage was not difficult – the bleeding was a little heavier than normal, like a strong period. I thought that this was because it was only an early pregnancy. As it started I hurt, as this was now my second chance gone, and again I was starting over.

Whilst the difference was that this time I had only a week of being and feeling pregnant, and I had little time to really get excited, it had brought back many of those memories from my first pregnancy. This time I worried that this could be a pattern, but put it aside. I now needed to focus on starting over again, letting my body heal, but also to stay focused on what could be in the future. This could be my age, but it could just be bad luck. I had to believe that there was still hope.

The entire process felt like such a rollercoaster ride, and I was back to starting a new cycle of conceiving. I hoped that my cycle would return to normal again quickly this time. After the first miscarriage it took almost three months to get my first period. I wasn't sure how patient I could be this time around, but what control did I really have over this? It was now a year since we started trying for a baby, and I was no further along. My April baby was no more, and the plans I had started to make had to be placed aside once again.

Although I was only pregnant a week, and for most of the week I was undergoing tests, for that one week I had hope. For a brief period of time, we had started to rebuild those dreams of being parents and holding that little baby that we wanted more than anything. We started revisiting our original plans of our baby and its future, and what we would be like as parents. It was the excitement and anticipation; this pregnancy took us by surprise and ended so very quickly after. But it was there, briefly, and now in that short space of time that hope was gone.

Help Not Needed

So after the second miscarriage we had many friends and family reinforce their support and love. Many were good sounding boards, empathetic and understanding, being there when we needed them. Sometimes we needed them, sometimes we didn't.

As some friends and family discovered our situation, there was the awkwardness, those who weren't sure what to say, how to respond, and those who just said the wrong things. I realised this was never intentional, but there were some comments that made it so much harder at times. Comments like, 'It will happen to you someday, you just need to be patient.' Thanks, I thought, that helps! Others like 'You deserve to be parents', 'It's just not your time this time', 'At least you can get pregnant' we heard several times, but they really didn't help much. In saying this however, we saw that many of our friends and family struggled with how to help us through the pain, and I understood that sometimes words don't mean how they sound.

My question is: 'What is the right thing to say to someone going through a miscarriage?' Having now been through two losses, would I know what to say to someone else? I really didn't know at this point. We are all different, and the reasons for miscarriages differ from woman to woman. We also had comments like: 'It wasn't meant to be,' and 'It's natures' way of making a decision.' True, but not helpful, however how can anyone say the right thing? 'I'm sorry' and 'I am here for you' were the best two statements anyone could have said to me at this time; that's all I wanted, just to know that they cared. Nothing can really make you feel better or solve the situation, but knowing that we had the support of family and friends helped us feel supported, when I felt everything else in my personal life was in complete havoc.

There were times when people around me talked about my miscarriages and I just wanted to scream, cry, throw a tantrum. Life could be so unfair! I truly felt that being pregnant and then not being pregnant was sending my poor body into turmoil and my emotions into disarray. I also realised that I couldn't close my feelings off or bottle them up, I needed a release.

Sometimes I just needed to be alone and let my thoughts, emotions and dreams wander. At times I would just dwell and grieve a loss of a baby that what never was, allow myself to think what could have been. That hurt, but it was my way of grieving. The other part of me would wish, dream and hope of what could be when that next pregnancy test showed positive.

It was also important for me and my husband to heal together, and appreciate that we were a strong couple who had a mountain of love for each other, and we would get through this, but it would take time.

As friends tried to help me move forward, I received many invitations for days and nights out, and sometimes that was the answer and sometimes I just wanted time on my own. I let myself, my body and mind decide what was right. I guess I became a little selfish, but it was my way of managing it. Sometimes the invites for nights out included cocktails and drinking (because, of course, I could eat and drink merrily now that I'm not pregnant). Sometimes this worked; often it was the pain I felt the morning after, with a large hangover, that didn't help me move forward. It was often a reminder of what was no longer. I really just needed my time, recovery of the mind and soul. Everyone copes differently and in their own way. There was no complete solution, but it was important to grieve and heal.

What I didn't need or want at that point was 'advice'. Advice on how to handle the situation, how I should or should not feel, what we should do next, or how we should approach the next pregnancy, was not helping either of us at that point in time.

I had many loved ones who suggested counselling, because talking to someone would, of course, make me feel better about losing two babies. I know now that this was my bitterness of what I had lost, and at the time I felt I had my own way of managing and dealing with that loss. I didn't feel ready to talk to anyone. I understood myself enough to know counselling wasn't the right type of help, and I would feel better focusing on the good things I had in my life, and to plan on moving forward once again.

Those of my friends who had unfortunately experienced miscarriages or struggles with pregnancy were also generous when offering their own advice, support and potential success stories. It was good to empathise, feel that you're not alone, and hear the stories of those who had been there, but now had their bouncy babies and success stories. Nonetheless, it was a difficult constant reminder that we didn't have our baby, and it was all so hard and just plain unfair. Two pregnancies, no baby, surely next time had to be our turn.

As our closest friends and family now knew, we were trying, and we clearly had the ability to get pregnant, twice in six months. There was also the anticipation that started building as they waited for the next 'time' and good news. I found myself halting before making statements that started with 'Guess what' or 'I have something to tell you' in general conversation, as suddenly the next words out of mouths of others were 'You're pregnant again?' and most of the time I was just going to tell them something exciting about my weekend. I had to closely manage the way I opened topics, as each time I heard those words it was a blunt reminder of what we had lost.

I also had to be careful what I wore as suddenly a floaty top may allude to me 'hiding a small tummy'. Even eating out had to be managed carefully. If I drove, hence didn't have a glass of wine, suddenly eyebrows raised and

I felt I was constantly justifying my actions or just over compensating for what was just not there.

I appreciate that some of the comments I've made in this chapter sound ungrateful, perhaps a little negative, but self-preservation was important during these times, for my own sanity. Sometimes I learnt that this meant being a little selfish and focusing on myself, my own feelings and my relationship with my husband. It was important to me that my husband and I stayed strong together, and we did not let this hurt how we felt about each other, and we loved each other dearly. My husband was my world and my strength. I found my best friend and my true soul mate in the man I married, and it was incredibly important to put that first above all else. We were going through this together.

Many times throughout the miscarriages we had, it occurred to me that my husband was forgotten. In fact, sometimes, I was lax in thinking how he was hurting too. There were times where I felt I did only think of my own physical and emotional pain, and I had to remind myself that he was also grieving, in many different ways to myself.

My husband didn't talk much to his own friends and family. I recognised that he tended to keep his feelings and thoughts to himself. Sometimes I wondered if he was protecting me, and I also realised that this was his way of coping with the loss we'd experienced. For me I recognised that talking to others did help me process what had happened; even just sharing the experience itself and how I felt was helpful. I wasn't looking for solutions; I just wanted my closest friends to listen and empathise. My family and friends were there for me when I needed them, and they helped, even if they didn't know it at the time.

As a couple we found opportunities for solace, taking time out and booking a weekend away – after everything, life does go on. We still maintained hope that our next pregnancy would happen soon, and that next time would be our time. That in itself was the one thing that helped us through this difficult time.

Social Enigma

The world of social media sometimes dumbfounds me. When I joined one of the most popular social networking pages, it was at a time when I was leaving my home country to work abroad. It was a great tool to stay in touch with family and friends, share my experiences and travels, and to just keep the connections alive. To be honest I'm terrible at staying in touch otherwise, and with time zone challenges, I would hardly ever phone my friends. Had it not been for the social media pages, I'm sure I would have lost touch with many of my friends as their lives took different paths. It also helped me in reconnecting with lost friends from school and university, rebuilding friendships that had been lost over the years, and bridging the distance of being so very far away at times from those who I wanted to remain close to. This is truly the magic of social media and where its value really comes into play.

I have, however, recently become more cautious of the tool, as it opens up a myriad of questions around privacy and sense of self discretion. Perhaps it's just me, but when did social media become the dumping ground for problems, or a showcase diary of every waking moment of our lives? I watch in awe and sometimes unease as people expose their innermost feelings, issues and every day challenges across the World Wide Web. You watch the break-ups and make-ups, the woes and rants, and those who respond become somewhat of an agony aunt to friends or connections that perhaps they only know through the online world.

I then see those ambiguous statements like: 'Sometimes I feel like giving up' or 'What's wrong with me?' and it makes me wonder, do people just not talk anymore? I feel like responding, stating the obvious: just pick up the phone and have a conversation! It's such an obvious cry for help or attention, seeking out responses of sympathy and support. I watch in wonder as I reflect on my own experiences, when things have been at their worst. Each to their own I guess, but personally, talking to a friend or a loved one for me is more immediate and comforting. It feels like human interaction is now missing and I fear we have in some ways isolated ourselves from actual conversation and connection. I know I am just uncomfortable with the concept of exposing myself so broadly and openly across an audience who will only view my problems or posts mixed across their own personal page alongside everyone else's.

Perhaps I'm taking a selfish view, but to be perfectly blunt on the topic, I really have no interest if someone is 'awake at two a.m., and cannot sleep', or that 'the car broke down this morning,' and you were 'late to work'.

When I read that traffic is chaos, a train is missed, or when it's pasta and chicken for dinner, I have to question when the online world became the first place to share a running commentary of the normal things that just happen in our daily lives. Pictures of food, the television screen, or worse, the 'trout pout' selfie that is taken in several different poses daily, profile pictures updated, capturing today's latest close up pucker mouth shot; I must be missing something here for sure. To be frank, it's never flattering to put a camera that close to anyone's face, yet it seems totally acceptable in the world of social media.

Then there are political, religious, social activist and animal rights posts, each making me cringe, as photos are spread across the pages, telling its audiences that if we don't share or comment we are inhumane. Yet people comment, share and encourage these posts, and you see them loop around continuously through different contacts and forums.

I do realise that in writing this chapter, I'm potentially dividing views on this particular controversial subject. There are those who will read this and potentially identify with my comments, or partially agree. Whether you have a social media page or not, everyone has their own view on the subject. Others reading this may question my motives, feel I'm making judgement, and question why I'm still active on social media or even link to friends who conduct themselves in ways I've just criticized. I accept that, and those who I am connected with today I value as friends, and they are the people I enjoy remaining in contact with. Whether I agree or disagree with any actions in the online world, I accept that we all have our own motives, and my views are my own sentiments, formed from my own experiences.

Having now dealt with two losses and some health issues along the way, I found it difficult at times watching others go through their day to day lives, highlighting problems that seemed to me quite trivial matters. Perhaps it was just me; I had become far more sensitive to these posts, irritated even at times. I felt that social media had become a forum to air dirty laundry or just complain. It also made me more conscious of my own posts, what I shared with others, and how something simple could easily offend or distress someone else that I may be connected with, even if to me it didn't seem consequential.

Watching others' pregnancy posts also started to become difficult. Month after month, I read new pregnancy announcements, each proudly showing their own little black and white scan photo, which would be posted as the latest profile picture. I'd see and read, day by day and month to month progress checks on pregnancies, pictures of growing bellies, and hear about habits, food, likes and dislikes. It was an exciting time for these expectant mums, and I certainly didn't begrudge them for anything. I just desperately wanted to be experiencing it all too, and reading every post and update was a constant reminder of what I had lost.

What was harder than anything was hearing the petty groans about being pregnant, being fat, tired or just going through some of the ups and downs that were to be expected as you grow a little human being inside you. Can't sleep, discomfort, fat ankles... it's not like any of this was a big surprise. Surely they did their homework before it all happened? I wanted those fat ankles, I wanted the heartburn. If this was the cross to bear, I would happily endure, if only to hold a happy, healthy baby at the other end. I started to 'unfollow' friends or hide their posts, as it started to upset me reading the posts that complained about sleepless nights, baby crying, breastfeeding, vomit, or toilet troubles. Each one felt like salt in an open wound, rubbing it in further, and to me, these were the sacrifices each parent made in that wonderful journey that was parenthood.

Don't get me wrong; I'm under no illusion that having a new born baby is an easy ride. In fact, many of my parent friends have given ample warnings on how hard it really is. Even then, knowing this, I realise both myself and my husband will be in for a shock when (and if) it really happens. Sleep deprivation, uncertainty, lack of control, and just being completely unaware of what to do in every situation parenthood throws your way – no amount of training or preparation will be enough. I know that! But surely the mothers' groups, support groups and 'real life friends' are the people you go to when you're lost? I just didn't want to read about it every day, how it was 'so tough', or that it was 'dull' and that life was now just about nappies, washing, cleaning, daytime television and waiting for the other half to return from work. With such terrible hardships in parenting, I should be so lucky, right? OK, now I'm the one grumbling, pot calling kettle black and all that. I guess what I'm saying here, is that nothing comes easy, and everyone has the right to grumble, but on these social media pages, it's there in the open for everyone to see and read, and it's hard to comprehend when there is no context given to statements for interpretation. Sometimes the people reading these posts are like me, someone who is suffering, wishing they could just have a chance to go through all these wonderful struggles themselves, and knowing this, I would be consciously sensitive when it is my time, on how I portray those challenges.

To be fair, it's not all bad in the world of social media. I love reading the good news stories; they give me hope for my own future and what it may hold. When I do see that first picture of a new born baby in its parent's arms, it's that look when they hold their child for the first time that cannot be forsaken. The obvious love, gratitude and relief, knowing that they have finally reached a point where that precious little baby is delivered healthy and happy. It is just such a precious time and should be celebrated. I see the moments captured such as birthdays, christenings and Christmas and how social media enables us to reach those who cannot be there in person, all across the world. This is what I truly love about the concept – the power of connection!

In a bizarre turn of events, I have started to see people use social media more so than with just a personal profile page; they are now setting up sub-sites for businesses, interests, pets and even have one in the name of their own new born child. It baffled me at the start, as these little ones were only months old, couldn't walk, talk, hardly communicate, let alone start building their own connections within the online community. It intrigued me as my friends, who were new parents, would start building their baby's online profile page, with photos, tagged events and even sending out friendship invitations to connect. I wasn't sure how I felt about being a friend to someone who could only gargle at this point of their life. Don't get me wrong, I adore their kids, but I really didn't see the purpose of a nearly forty year old and a baby four months old, being linked. Really? What would they care what holiday plans I'm making for this summer?

In time, however, having reflected on this, I'd come to a realisation that what these parents were actually doing was quite smart, ingenious even. You see, my mother kept sequential photo albums from the day I was born, and all throughout my childhood, teenage and adult years. She was meticulous and dedicated to maintaining these, noting key events, dates, ages, and ensuring that each photo was labelled, naming everyone included in the picture, so that in time, I could look back at the memories and see my life progress on these wonderful pages she had so lovingly created. My mother has shelves of these albums, and they sit in her home waiting for someone to pick them up one by one, appreciating the effort and devotion that that has gone into each one. Some of the photos are faded, and the albums are sometimes a little stiff due to their age, but they are always there waiting for me if ever I have a question about a time and place, or just feel like taking a trip down memory lane to cringe at some of the trends or hairstyles of that era.

Honestly, my mother must have spent hours taking photos, getting them processed (in the days of processed film), planning each album and writing commentary beside each picture. Some may feel that it's a waste of time, that these old relics will just gather dust, never to be truly appreciated. For me it's a wonderful picture diary of my growing up, of friends and relatives, those here still today and those who are now gone but forever in my heart. I'd spend hours sometimes just trawling through the memories, smiling, sometimes shuddering, as I would look at myself throughout the years, and would privately thank my mum for keeping such an incredible record of my own personal history.

Where am I going with this? Well, these parents, my friends, in setting up their child's online profile, have in fact done the exact same thing that my mother started all those years ago, but in a much more efficient way. The online world is a wonderful beast for some things, and this is where social media really plays its part. These parents have in fact set up an online sequential album for each of their own children from the day of birth. Setting up individualised profile pages has enabled them to capture every photo, tagged with dates and commentary, keeping a precise 'to the moment' record of their baby's growth and development, every special event, holiday and outing. It's now all in one place that can be accessed by all family and friends, at any time and anywhere in the world. It can never be destroyed by fire, lost or stolen, and the photos won't fade. It's there, and it's available, and one day those children can look back in time, with the click of a mouse.

So have the days of clunky albums with their plastic sleeves and taped in photos gone forever? Right now I'm not sure, but perhaps it's heading that way. I guess there are pros and cons for both, and I wonder whether the online pages created can really replace the love and effort that went into those old albums my mother created all those years ago. I love the thought of book shelves filled with old dated albums passed on through my own generations, but yet in reality, with so much technology, the concept starts to feel dated. Perhaps there is room in this world for both?

Whilst initially the thought of creating a page for a new born baby seemed a little crazy to me, I've recognised that it's a valuable and efficient way to store memories and moments. Particularly when those moments move so fast, time elapses, and it feels as though you can blink and those little babies are grown up already. What would I do if I ever had the chance to have a baby of my own? I'm not sure to be honest. Social media, for all its good and its flaws, is a great connection tool. Whilst my views can potentially be controversial and even critical at times, I see the value in what it offers, and how I've been able to use it to share and build on friendships. Whilst I'll never totally agree with how it's used in some forums, that is my own issue and no one else's, and that's okay.

'Tis the Season

I had reconciled to myself by November that if we didn't fall pregnant again in the next cycle, I would enjoy the festive season for all the celebrations and indulgences it offers.

It's like everything in life – if you want something so much, it's all you can think about. You make plans and you dream of a future that seems so straight forward in your head, and then when things go wrong, suddenly your path changes and your plans alter. Just as you become content, reconciled with that alternative, the path changes again. That's life, I guess.

After our second miscarriage, I felt as though my whole life revolved around cycles, ovulating, pregnancy tests and timed sex. It was ruling my very existence, my every thought, and I started to stop planning other things in my life, making decisions around a 'potential pregnancy' that may never be. I don't even know if my husband was aware how much the entire process took up every thought of every day, and when I tried to explain it to him, he suggested that I stop thinking about it all the time. Not the easiest suggestion to agree to but he was right. I had to find a way to start living my life again, stop the forever planning and thinking.

I made the decision to throw away all of my ovulation tests, remove any applications from my mobile phone and iPad, and just stop looking at calendar dates, website forums or any other materials that would get me thinking about my options. I had to believe that what will be, will be. Our relationship was too important to keep this up, it started to feel robotic, and we needed to bring that spontaneity back, plan holidays and just have fun. It wasn't easy, and of course I still thought about pregnancy often, as I knew we were throwing chance to the wind in not measuring cycles or following specific timings, but it was also important for my own sanity to just step back and let nature take its course.

Like the second pregnancy, I knew I was pregnant before I tested. I was at work and it was three months after the second miscarriage. I was attending a training session with many of my colleagues, and I felt uncomfortable, feeling myself getting restless just sitting and listening to the facilitator. It was that familiar abdominal pull, not cramping, just tightness, like I needed to stand up and stretch or walk around. I felt strange, and I realised that this was more than just a pre-period cramp.

It was two weeks before our Christmas break and I was able to finish work early, so I picked up a test on the way home from work that day. However, I didn't test that night. Again I left it, telling myself I needed to be absolutely sure. The next morning I was positive that I was pregnant; that same feeling in my lower abdomen was still there. Along with that, my boobs were tender and I felt quite fatigued in general. I hadn't really been watching my cycle, but I knew my period was due around the weekend from looking back through my diary. I didn't know the exact date, but that seemed about right. I did know that this was too familiar a feeling to ignore. So I tested.

As I watched and waited for the test result to appear, I was nervous once again. When the word 'pregnant' appeared I was taken back. I'm not sure why. Whilst I had felt that this was it, and I was confident I was pregnant, there is always a strange feeling or response when you actually see those words appear the first time in your cycle. That response hits you in the heart, it's the hope and the anticipation, but this time it was also the fear, fear of going through another loss again. I stopped myself from heading down that path. It had to be right this time; it had to be our time. My gut feeling said that we would have our 'rainbow baby' this time and it would be a healthy pregnancy. I was positive.

Christmas parties and celebrations were difficult, particularly as I'm known to enjoy a glass of bubbly, especially on festive occasions. I became an artist in 'faking it', keeping a glass of drink in hand all night, finding opportunities to tip it out slightly so it looked as though it was depleting, putting the drink to my lips as though to have a sip, refilling it at obvious locations. I wasn't taking any chances, but I also didn't want my colleagues and acquaintances to start guessing at such an early stage of our pregnancy.

I only had two weeks of keeping up this performance, and then my husband and I were on annual leave for the Christmas period. We were going away for Christmas to the New Forest with my brother; his wife, who was almost eight months' pregnant; and my gorgeous three-year-old nephew and godson. It was a perfect way to spend Christmas, in a small cottage in the serene countryside, where we could enjoy our festive celebrations.

Watching my sister-in-law revel in her final months of pregnancy was lovely and encouraging. Her second pregnancy had unfortunately resulted in a missed miscarriage, no heartbeat at their first scan. It was devastating and this was such a shock after she'd had such a very healthy pregnancy with her first son, my gorgeous nephew.

This, my now third pregnancy was my hope! I had gone through two miscarriages in the year gone, and this pregnancy was the one! Clearly we had no issue getting pregnant, and in fact we realised how lucky we actually were when we heard stories of friends who had been trying for months, sometimes years. Three pregnancies in one year, surely this had to be our time now. All the dates felt like they were lining up nicely, with our due date late August, closer to my birthday.

This pregnancy also felt right. From the moment I thought I was pregnant until the test, it felt different, more promising, and I felt confident that things would go well for us this time. We had gone through too much, come too far, hurt so much. This was, after all, the festive season, and we had something to feel truly festive about.

All negative thoughts I put away to the back of my mind and I focused on the moment, having fun just being excited alongside my pregnant sister-in-law, knowing we would have new born babies six months apart. It was going to be a happy Christmas, or so I kept telling myself.

Bah Humbug

We had to know it would be too good to be true! Two days before Christmas day, I went to the bathroom of the small cottage we were renting, and there was blood. Not a lot but enough to send my heart racing, take the breath from my mouth, and make my world spin.

'*Not again*!' I cried mournfully. I felt my chest constrict and I leant back against the small bathroom wall whilst I composed myself. I started to cry with fear, I couldn't do this again. I wiped to find a little more blood; it was brownish in colour and looked old but it was still blood. I didn't know what it meant but my oblivious dream of a smooth pregnancy suddenly crash landed.

I was glad to have my husband, my brother and my sister-in-law there with me, to support and keep me positive. They calmed me, assured me that I should not worry, panic, and stress myself. Hard not to, but I nodded as they all repeated the same thing together. A lot of people get breakthrough bleeding in early pregnancy; these stories were all online with a very healthy baby as a result. The assurances were helpful, but didn't send that small essence of doubt away. I, of course, jumped on Google, where I found many success stories to help reassure me, but an equal number of stories that kept me worried.

It was also helpful having my spirited three year old nephew in the house. With his energy and excitement around Christmas, Santa arriving and the mountain of presents under our makeshift holiday tree with his name on most of them, I really couldn't stay negative or dwell in my worries.

There is nothing more brilliant than seeing Christmas through a child's eyes. This year was really the first year that my nephew seemed to truly understand Christmas, well, in the way a young child can understand it. Christmas for kids is about Santa and reindeers, decorating the house, lots of sweets and treats, and of course presents under the tree. How could I not get excited about such an amazing time of year?

I kept thinking, hoping that this time next year there would be two more little ones to enjoy Christmas with, another nephew almost one, and my little one who would be barely four months old. That would be wonderful.

The bleeding was sparse, and it remained on and off over Christmas, Boxing Day and for the rest of our small vacation. Sometimes it would disappear for hours, and then just return with a few spots. I'd forget about it, enjoy the festive activities, and then going to the bathroom would send me a blunt reminder, driving me to question whether I was setting myself up for another fall with this pregnancy.

We had a scan booked on December 30th, for our return from the New Forest, and it would hopefully reassure us that all was well and we were growing a healthy little baby. By then I would be just over six weeks, so surely they would see a heartbeat.

We were leaving for Ireland on the 31st December, and we were hoping to bring my husband's parents some good news of pending grandparenthood, showing them the evidence in a little black and white scan photo. That was our plan.

New Year, New Hope...

The scan didn't give us hope unfortunately. My husband and I had booked and paid for this scan privately, as we wanted to get early reassurance. It would be worth it, and given our history with early pregnancy loss I was not going to wait until thirteen weeks, I just couldn't.

Well, the sonographer asked me my dates, putting me at just over six weeks. She explained that we should see a heartbeat but did prepare us that not all pregnancies were the same. She was managing our expectations.

When she started the scan, she immediately saw the pregnancy, and stated so. My heart was beating so fast and I held my husband's hand tightly. She hesitated.

'It isn't dating at six weeks,' she said calmly, 'I am measuring just over five and half weeks.'

'What does that mean?' I jumped in. Was this good or bad news? I couldn't read her face.

'I can see a pregnancy sac, and a foetal pole, but no heartbeat. It could be that you got your dates wrong, or you ovulated later than you thought. I normally suggest a follow up scan in a week's time to check the pregnancy is progressing,' she explained to both of us.

I slowly processed what she had said, so it wasn't bad news, perhaps it was almost a week behind. My dates couldn't be wrong, could they? Maybe they were? I wasn't really tracking this pregnancy, my cycle. I must have it all wrong. That's good. At least it's not too far out. It's just a slow grower. All these thoughts were soaring through my head.

I dressed and then followed my husband out of the room. She reassured me that it was just an early scan, and that often it's very hard to tell at this stage, as the baby is only a millimetre long. That calmed me a little.

'I'm positive; I'm not worried at all.' My husband's statement to me as we walked to the car brought me out of my trance of a million conflicting thoughts.

'OK, me neither,' I responded, rather unconvincingly, I'd suggest. He squeezed my hand encouragingly. We were heading to Ireland the next day, and this was good news. I could book the follow up scan for our return the next week, and in the meantime we could just enjoy the New Year, and time with family and friends in Ireland!

In the meantime I would follow all the rules, do everything right, and give this baby every chance to grow and develop inside me. There was still hope!

We had a quiet but homely New Year's celebration with another couple on the north coast of Ireland. We saw the midnight countdown in an apartment overlooking the sea, with a glass frontage and a warming fireplace. My husband and his friends enjoyed many a glass of champagne, whilst I suitably drank non-alcoholic bubbly (in a champagne glass of course). It was entertaining watching them get a little tiddly as the night went on, and I was content being the spectator. It was fun staying up until the early hours of the morning, indulging in treats and savoury snacks, and playing board games until our eyes were stinging from tiredness. It was low key but it was a great way to see the New Year in. My husband and I toasted to our future, staying hopeful for the year ahead.

The next few days were spent with family in Ireland and it felt right to share our news with them, always giving the proviso that we were awaiting a follow up scan but we hoping for a positive result. It was lovely to share the excitement and the anticipation, but when it was time to go home, we were again reminded of the reality of our situation. There were still three more days until our follow up scan; it was just a waiting game now and time felt like it stood still as each day seemed to drag its heels.

The day of the scan arrived again, and I felt like I was experiencing déjà vu! I felt my stomach lurch, like I was going to be ill, as we walked up that familiar corridor, back through the hospital that had managed our first two miscarriages. In that sonographer's office again, I willed myself to stay positive. Having had two negative experiences, I kept telling myself everything would be fine, I just needed to hear that the baby had grown since last time, and for them to see the heart beating strongly. At just over seven weeks, there should certainly be a heartbeat now.

There was no heartbeat. My whole body went numb and I was heartbroken as the sonographer told us the news. The pregnancy was still only measuring just on six weeks, it had barely grown at all and it was happening again. I had known this in my heart before the outcome of the scan.

Because the first scan was done privately, I heard her explain to me and my husband that there needed to be another follow up scan in seven days to confirm miscarriage. I heard that it wasn't hopeful, that I may start miscarrying normally. They were just voices and echoes in my head, it felt surreal. Everything was crumbling around me; that hurt, the pain and the grief I'd experienced before were suddenly flooding back in again. This time it felt worse. Was it? I couldn't remember. Tears flooded down my face, my breathing was jagged, I did all I could to control myself from just losing it completely.

My husband held me and he walked me out of the hospital. I sat in the passenger seat in tears as he drove me home. Every now and then he would just softly place his palm on my leg. He felt helpless, he was hurting too. Three losses in twelve months, hadn't we been through enough? How do you move forward from here? My mind was clouded in grief and sadness and it was too hard to see a way out of it. I didn't know if I could get through it this time; it enveloped me.

I was supposed to be in the office for the rest of the afternoon, but I couldn't even fathom being around anyone right now. When we arrived home, I switched my computer on with the intention to work, but all I could do was just sit there staring blankly at the screen, my eyes welling with tears and my mind just a blur. I'm not sure how long I sat there before I realised that I just needed to curl up in bed and switch off from the world altogether. The worst part was knowing that this wasn't over. I still had to wait seven days to go back to that dark room, to be re-scanned, with the knowledge that this pregnancy was over. I was also conscious that my body had not yet experienced any physical signs of the miscarriage, and I had no idea when I could expect that to begin. I really wasn't sure how I would get through the next few hours let alone another week. My world had just fallen apart once again.

The Foolish Martyr

Luckily I didn't need to wait a week. Two days after my scan, the miscarriage started. Whilst I would have preferred surgical removal again, I was a little relieved that I didn't need to wait for the third scan and go through that entire process of setting up the surgical appointment. I hoped that it would be quick and over with and I could just get on with life.

I had returned to work on that day it started – my mind had been less clouded with grief and I needed the distraction to be honest. Sitting at home, dwelling on my own misery wasn't helping, and sometimes it's just easier to carry on with tasks and put the entire ordeal out of mind. I telephoned the hospital and cancelled my scheduled scan. The nurse on duty agreed that there was no point coming in, and advised me to contact the hospital if my bleeding got too heavy or I started to feel unwell. The arrangement worked for me, and I decided to treat this as just a very strong period that may last around a week.

The cramping was quite strong, very painful at times, and the bleeding was heavy, much heavier than I'd experienced previously. I kept waiting for it to lighten, to start slowing down, but it didn't. Work was also incredibly busy, so I had limited time to over think about what my body was going through or to dwell on the grief. To be honest, on reflection, I just wanted to ignore it, put it to the back of my mind, and carry on with other things so that I could keep going. Sitting still with time on my own brought back the flood of emotions, and I didn't want to deal with that.

I was scheduled to travel with work for a two-day conference to Poland, just three weeks after I had started the miscarriage. The bleeding and pain had continued, and it was constant, but it hadn't worsened. I had a fairly quiet weekend before the conference, and whilst I felt generally fatigued and sore, I was on regular low dose pain killers to keep the pain at bay. I was on the early morning, red eye flight to Poland, and I'd left the house at five a.m. I never sleep on flights, not even long haul flights. I'm not sure why, but even with years of flying I've never really mastered it. However, on this early morning journey I found it hard to keep my eyes open, and I must have had at least a good two hours' sleep on the inbound journey. My body clearly needed it! I knew I looked like a wreck but life goes on, and I couldn't just halt everything waiting for this miscarriage to finish. Two weeks in and there were no apparent signs yet of it stopping.

During the conference, I was to facilitate an afternoon workshop session. Training, facilitation and presentations are a part of the job that I really enjoy, and I was actually looking forward to this. For a couple of hours, I wanted to just focus all my energy and passion into a group of leaders, and just play my role in bringing them together for a common cause. I was in the zone and about three quarters of the way through the session when I felt a little faint, and a hot flush ran through me. I also felt something else and needed to run to the bathroom. I asked the group to work on some ideas on their own, and rushed off.

I went to the bathroom and checked my underwear. The pad I had been wearing was soaked through with sizeable clots. I wiped and my hand filled with more blood. I sat on the toilet quickly, and watched between my legs as a downpour of blood filled the bowl. I hadn't brought a pad to change with me, and my underwear was stained. I checked my trousers and I was thankful I'd decided to wear black that day. They had a small spot, but I'd caught it in time. I felt drained and worried, being in another country, not knowing if this would continue, get heavier, or worse. I had an hour left of this workshop and I couldn't just walk out now. I packed toilet paper into my pants to temporarily replace my pad, but I needed to get to my suitcase to replace that quickly. I composed myself and went back into the workshop room.

I looked at my own agenda and quickly reshuffled, calling a fifteen minute break, which would allow me to fix myself up properly. Once I had replaced the pad, I felt calmer, more in control. I tailored the workshop to allow general thinking and discussion time for the attendees, which allowed me to head to the bathroom to check myself periodically. I was meant to attend dinner that night with the group, but I made some polite apologies and went straight to the hotel room. I felt terrible! I just needed to order some light room service, sleep and look forward to heading home the next day.

I was not well the next day at all, still experiencing more bleeding and pain, and I just didn't feel good in general. I sat through the conference meeting but I really don't recall much of the conversation points. I was to leave by three p.m. for my flight, and I wouldn't arrive home in my bed until around eleven p.m that night. Whilst normally travel didn't bother me, I really did not feel up to waiting around in airport terminals, or sitting on a cramped flight. I just wanted the comfort of my home and my bed.

My husband and I are often passing ships in the night. He was asleep when I got home and I didn't wake him. I literally dropped my suitcase and crept into bed. I don't even recall my head hitting the pillow. My body must have been so exhausted, as I cannot even remember him leaving in the morning. My husband always sets his alarms early, and that morning was no exception as he was scheduled to travel to one of his regional offices for the day. He wouldn't be home until late that evening. There wasn't even the chance to update him on my past few days.

I could barely move when I woke later that morning, and I succumbed to a day in bed, as I couldn't even fathom getting myself dressed, let alone spending a day in the office. I sent a text through to my team and my manager, and just closed my eyes again. I wasn't sure what I had planned for work that day, or what was in my calendar. I was too unwell to even worry about it. That's not like me.

I'm not sure how long I slept but when I woke I was shivering, like my entire body was freezing. My entire body was uncontrollably convulsing, and I felt extremely cold all over. I pulled the blankets up and turned my electric blanket up, but the shivering wouldn't stop. I crawled across the bed, barely being able to control my body, and gulped down the bottle of water, spilling it over the bed, as my teeth continued to chatter wildly. My chest was heaving by this stage, and I started to panic. I couldn't stand up; I could hardly control any of my limbs. I wrapped more of the blanket around me and rubbed my arms and my legs vigorously trying to control my body's reaction. This wasn't a normal reaction to cold weather, this was something else!

So yes, I admit wholeheartedly that I had been a little silly going back to work so quickly, agreeing to an overseas work conference, and generally ignoring the many help signals my body had been sending. I was poorly, and I needed to take some action here. I realised that my body was reacting, and that this was not a normal miscarriage. I was now quite frightened. Reflecting on what had happened, I realise my ignorance and quest to carry on as normal was stupid, but it was my way of dealing with the pain and loss I had experienced. I needed to feel like my life would return to normal again, and so I failed to take heed of the signals my body was sending me and what I was actually experiencing, or just accept that actually something was not OK here.

Many people asked me why I didn't stop or take heed at the time. The answer is not even clear to me. People deal with grief differently, and my only excuse was that I was trying to move on from the pain in the only way I knew how.

When my body finally calmed, I called the local doctor's surgery. My doctor called me back an hour later, and as I explained what was happening she chastised me also for ignoring what I'd been experiencing. She said it sounded as though I had a blood infection and I would need to get to the hospital immediately for examination and antibiotics. As I was home alone I had no choice but to wait for my husband to arrive home.

I had two more episodes of these frightening convulsions that day, on my own, and each time I grew more and more frightened. Each time, I couldn't do a thing; I had to wait them out, and when they calmed down after five minutes, I felt OK again. I wondered if I should call the hospital or an ambulance, but then it seemed frivolous and unnecessary when it was all over.

It was late when my husband did arrive home that night, and needless to say he was also upset at me for doing nothing, not calling the ambulance, not calling him. I was tired and I had needed rest and sleep, and I tried to explain that there was nothing he could have done at the time. He tried to convince me to head to the hospital late that evening, and I assured him that if I experienced another convulsion I would. I'd also not eaten a proper meal, so he cooked me up something healthy and hearty, and sat with me, ensuring I ate every last bite. We agreed to go to the hospital first thing in the morning, and that night I slept soundly with no further episodes.

Hospital Yo-Yo

We went to the hospital the next morning, and the doctor gave me some antibiotics to rid my body of any infection and hopefully ensure that I'd have no further convulsions or shaking episodes. Another scan was scheduled to see what was happening with the miscarriage, and I was sent back down to the early pregnancy unit. My husband and I sat there in the waiting lounge with lots of excited expectant parents around us. I looked ragged, pale and miserable, and stood out like a sore thumb amongst the others seated around me. It seemed such an injustice, as we sat outside that early scan room, waiting and just watching every other couple enter and then leave, holding their small black and white scan photos, excited with their own prospects of starting a family. After what seemed an eternity, we were called into that small room again, that room that had brought me nothing but bad news each time.

'I'm not sure why they have sent you here,' grumbled the sonographer. She wasn't the same woman I had last time I was here. Honestly how would I know why they sent me here? Why the hell was she asking me? I'd have honestly preferred not to come back to this room, knowing that this was the place that crushed my hopes over three weeks ago.

'We only do early pregnancy scans,' she continued to inform me, like it was my decision to be in this claustrophobic room again. She looked at me for a response – what was I to say? I was so tired and sick; my brain wasn't really functioning quickly, and I was half naked, on the table just waiting for the scan to be over with, waiting to find out what was wrong so I could go back home to bed to sleep.

'I have no idea, ask the doctor.' I couldn't care either way. Just send me home, I thought.

'Well I'm not sure what I can tell you!' this woman was getting on my nerves now. She started looking at the screen as she did the internal scan. I just put my head back and closed my eyes; there wasn't anything hopeful in this encounter with the sonographer, and all I wanted was to find out what was wrong and get this miscarriage over with. 'Well, there's still retained products in there, so you'll continue to experience bleeding until its gone, or you may stop bleeding and have an extra heavy period. That's all I can tell you.' I was asked to get up and get dressed and wait for a consultant. They sat me again outside the waiting room.

For over an hour I sat there waiting. My husband joined me, sitting beside me, holding my hand and stroking my palm in support. I lay my head on his shoulder, wishing this all to go away. All the while this torture continued as we watched more parents go in and out for their scan appointment, hearing the excitement before the scan and watching them exit the little room with beaming smiles on their faces. I looked like death, and they must have wondered what we were doing, and why this pale, glum woman was just sitting there. I just wanted to scream, but even if I tried I'm not sure I had the energy to release more than a squeak.

Finally I'd had enough; I waited for one of the nurses to appear, and I stated my case, asked how much longer, and why I had to sit here just watching and waiting. I was upset, teary, tired and just in a whole lot of pain. She sympathised with me and led both of us to a separate room to wait; she assured us that the consultant was on her way, and would see me soon. Another thirty minutes passed, and finally the door opened. The consultant looked quite young, and she was holding my now very thick hospital file. She sat down in the chair in front of us and turned to me with a sympathetic look, 'So you are miscarrying, I'm sorry for your sad news. There is not much you can do but just wait it out,' she informed us. I was confused.

'Yes I know I'm miscarrying,' I started calmly, trying to hold my emotions. 'I've been bleeding for over three weeks, and really heavily, and I'm in lots of pain.' I was trying to explain my situation but it was so hard, the words just weren't coming out the way I wanted them to.

'Yes unfortunately, you will miscarry all of the retained products in your womb. There's still some left. You will continue to naturally miscarry until that's over.

124

I'm sorry to hear of your miscarriage.' She sounded like a robot, like this was her standard speech.

'Have you read my file?' Surely she knew my history, what had happened.

'No not all of it. I've read the results of the scan you've just had,' she explained.

'I've been bleeding for over three weeks, I'm so sick. I'm in pain. I've had shivers. I'm on antibiotics.' I was talking in short sentences, trying to explain.

'She's not been well, she was sent here because she was having a shivering attack, by her GP,' my husband tried to explain but it was difficult for him, as he hadn't been there, and was only relaying what I'd told him.

'Yes, well there is nothing I can really prescribe you, as you are having a natural miscarriage.' That was it! Her last statement, her whole demeanour seemed so indifferent to my situation. My emotions got the better of me.

'I know I'm miscarrying! That's not news to us, the baby's dead, and I know I'm losing it!' My voice raised, I started to cry. She hadn't even read my file, she was just ticking a box; she hadn't offered any help or any solutions! I stood up. 'You clearly can't help. You can't even be bothered to read the file.' I stormed out of the room and out of the hospital. I was crying so hard and I didn't care, I just wanted to go home! My husband chased after me, catching up with me as I reached the car park. He slowed me down, put his arm around me, and we walked.

'I'm so sorry!' I wailed. 'I embarrassed you.'

'You didn't embarrass me,' he was reassuring and I knew he understood my frustration.

'She couldn't even take time to read the file!' I was so angry.

'So what do you want to do? You really need to be seen by someone.' He didn't want to push me to go back in there, but he was worried.

'I have my antibiotics, I'll take them. I just want to go home and sleep.' Maybe that wasn't the best solution, but it was the only solution for me right now. The hospital system had not offered my any better alternatives. As we drove home, I started to feel guilty about my behaviour in the hospital. I had stormed out, and perhaps that wasn't the best solution to help me sort myself out.

'I'm going to call them back,' I told my husband, who just nodded in support and reached across to squeeze my hand. I dialled the early pregnancy unit and one of the nurses picked up the phone. I was still crying, so I must have sounded emotional, erratic. When I said my name, the nurse recognised me and said that the consultant had told her what had happened. I just cried again, explaining that I was so frustrated, that the consultant hadn't even read my notes. Instead, she just kept telling me I was miscarrying. I could hear in the tone of her response that she understood. She asked if I'd like to come back, see a different consultant. We were almost home and I just wanted to rest. I told her I couldn't be there again, in that unit with all those expectant mums going in and out, I just needed to rest and sleep. I was so tired, in pain, and just

126

over the entire experience. She reluctantly agreed, and advised me that I should go home, sleep and take my antibiotics, but if anything worsened I was to come back to accident and emergency immediately.

The antibiotics seemed to prevent further episodes of shivering and convulsions, but the bleeding continued and it remained heavy. I was tired, wiped out. I wasn't sure how much more blood I could actually keep losing, but it just didn't seem to be slowing down.

Over a week later, the bleeding started to become even heavier again. I hadn't wanted to raise concerns to my husband; I had been monitoring it closely but didn't want to cause alarm or further worry. However, on the Sunday evening I woke in the late hours of the night and felt it. I rushed to the bathroom, and the only way I can describe it is like turning on a tap. The blood rushed out as I sat there, and I could only watch it in horror, not sure what to do next.

When it felt like the rush had stopped I fixed myself up, and woke my husband. We called the hospital and were advised to come in immediately. The bleeding stayed heavy, and I was replacing my sanitary pad every ten to fifteen minutes. I was admitted into hospital and taken to a hospital ward, where they placed me on a drip to keep my fluids up, and administered all sorts of medications and injections to stop the bleeding and any infection. The amount of blood I was losing had concerned them and I was now being monitored closely.

Thankfully the medicines helped and it slowed quickly after that. Whilst I continued to show signs of miscarriage throughout the following weeks, it was now finally starting to improve day by day. Needless to say that this particular loss was not only emotionally draining, it was physically horrendous. I couldn't imagine starting over again at that point; in fact I knew I needed a break from it all. I was exhausted from the physical strain I had been through, my body felt wrecked, and I just felt flat and empty. After all of that, I still lost our third baby, our third opportunity to be a family. Each time it sprung to mind, I felt hopeless thinking that there must be something stopping us from getting pregnant. I knew I needed to find out some answers, given now we were officially classified as having 'recurrent miscarriage'. When I looked that up, most reference articles cite that only one percent of the female population experience recurrent miscarriage (three miscarriages in a row). Like most, the 'why us', and 'what are we doing wrong' questions came to mind, but in essence there isn't much you can do if you keep looking back, you can only move forward.

My husband even felt the heaviness of the entire ordeal, and he certainly didn't want to put me through the process again without some help. It scared him a great deal, seeing how quickly my body almost shut down, and how it had impacted me emotionally. We agreed to see a fertility specialist, even just as a first level consultation. It would help us decide what we could do from there.

Everyone is Expecting

I was always told that when you suddenly start taking an interest in something different, you notice everyone around you doing the same thing. Same goes for when you buy a new car or a new dress, suddenly you notice others who are wearing that same dress, or driving that same car. Silly analogy I know, but it really felt like that when we were going through our miscarriages.

All of a sudden it felt like everyone was getting pregnant, and when I went through that last miscarriage, I must have had several friends announce the arrival of their new born babies. Perhaps it's my age group, my friendship circles or just me being more aware of these scenarios all around me, but it did feel like babies were everywhere for that period in time.

It was those moments when I was feeling the most ill, depressed and just generally disappointed in our fate that I felt that it may never work out for us. It is those moments where you do start to feel sorry for yourself about what you don't have. Please don't misunderstand me, I was never resentful, and I was always very happy for others having success in their pregnancy journeys. I just wanted to be joining them in my own.

In fact I was more than excited to hear the very happy news that my brother and sister-in-law had given birth to a gorgeous bouncy little boy in early February. Yes, that was at the same time I was experiencing the worst part of my miscarriage, but it encouraged me to step out of that grey cloud I was hiding under at the time. This gorgeous little bub was my second nephew and another little bouncy ball of love I could spoil silly. We were sent the first pictures of that gorgeous little baby when he first entered the world, and were so very appreciative of being part of such an amazing moment. I couldn't wait to see him in person, hold him, and celebrate with my family a brilliant and amazing new arrival.

As I did sometimes look up the online forums for other women who were in my position, I watched comments where some women found it difficult to be around others who were pregnant, or they found it difficult to feel happiness for those who were having babies. Some even lost friendships over it, feeling that they could no longer be around their pregnant friends. I found this incredibly sad, that a friendship of many years could be lost so quickly, and I vowed this wouldn't be me. We each have our own coping mechanism, and I cannot judge others in their responses or whether this was right or wrong. Every person has their own coping mechanism, and it's about retaining your own sanity.

I guess what I am saying is that each time someone did announce a new pregnancy, or there was a new birth announcement, it did make for a solemn reminder of the loss we'd experienced. But then, at the same time, it also provided us with hope of something that could be, a dream we could one day realise.

I'm not saying it's easy! In fact it has been incredibly hard at times to stay positive, and keep a mindset that didn't just focus on the negatives. It would have been very easy to remain sad and feel sorry for myself. It was at those moments that I felt I was spiralling downwards – that I needed to keep reminding myself of what we did have in life, and what I should be grateful for. My husband was also very good at picking me up when I was particularly down. Life goes on, and the road certainly wasn't over, we may just need to take an alternative route to get there. I was determined to find a way forward, and I was hopeful that this fertility specialist may provide us with a solution.

In the Good Ol' Days....

It's funny when you speak to your mother or anyone of an older generation about pregnancy and loss. Particularly as nowadays technology and advancements in understanding pregnancy have improved immensely and continue to do so. Even in the past two years I've noticed the difference in tests and options available to newly pregnant mums.

Of course I had been confiding in my mum about our miscarriages, the challenges we were experiencing and most recently what we had been through. She found it difficult to relate, as she had never experienced miscarriage. She had three healthy children, each four years apart, although she often told me it took her a long time to conceive each. For her, hearing of our struggles was hard, and I know I'd often get upset over the phone, with her struggling to say the right things at the right time. She didn't know what to say to be honest, how could she? So we would often just talk in general about getting pregnant and what it was like in her time.

In the days when she was trying, almost forty years ago now, there were no ovulation tests, early pregnancy tests or applications to track your cycle times or calculate conception dates. It was all manual, generally based on good timing and a bit of temperature checking. Would that have been easier? Perhaps not knowing is more helpful. She'd often tell me that she would leave it to luck and then just wait until she was two weeks late from her period before even going to see the doctor. It was then that the doctor himself would administer a pregnancy test, and she would get her results from there. I knew how impatient I had been; I could barely hold out until my period was due, and often in the early days of trying, I'd start testing four or five days before my cycle due date.

There was limited information available, and certainly no Internet, so many times Mum was alone in the process, just waiting and wondering. There were of course reference books, but no online forums or chat boards, to seek out immediate answers (right or wrong), or just to connect with others going through the same situation.

My mum also told me that sometimes when her period was late, she'd get her hopes up, and it would then arrive a week or two later; sometimes she would have a six or seven week cycle. She told me that she sometimes had irregular cycles, particularly when she was trying to conceive, and that these would often result in a heavier period. We both talked at length, and we'd often wondered if these had potentially been an early pregnancy that hadn't been viable. In those times I guess you wouldn't know for sure.

My mother-in-law also had a similar story, although she had unfortunately experienced a miscarriage when she was younger. Again, she wouldn't go to her doctor for tests until six or seven weeks into a pregnancy, and where she lived, she would have to wait sometimes a week for the result. I can't imagine the anxiety and hope that people must have experienced in those days waiting for the doctor to call them, whilst being sure it must be a positive result, as their period hadn't yet arrived.

In my mum's stories, she would also share that once she had her positive pregnancy result, there was very little in the way of knowledge and technology to really understand how her pregnancy was progressing. There were no early scans, just waiting and hoping that baby would grow and develop. She would, of course, have periodic check-ups with her general practitioner and consultant, and the heartbeat would be monitored once it could be heard through a stethoscope. However, the idea of seeing your baby inside with a scan was something she was truly envious of in today's world of technology. The concept of watching your little baby move inside you, to see its limbs and features, and discover whether it would be a boy or a girl was literally magical to her.

The availability of technology and testing made me grateful of our own situation. Even if I got past that first heartbeat, and was able to progress our pregnancy through the first trimester, I know for sure that I'd want the support of that technology along the way. I would want regular scans to reassure me throughout the pregnancy and I would want to undergo testing to ensure that the baby was healthy.

Perhaps there is an argument that knowing less in the early stages of pregnancy would reduce the stress and anxiety experienced just through sheer worrying. If I found out I was pregnant and could do nothing much more about it except wait with no technology to monitor the progress, would I have worked myself up into such a panic each time? Probably not. However, after multiple miscarriages I'm sure I would still have the worry and the fear – that will never disappear. I don't believe the outcome would have been any different either way, and I do believe I'd still be here today talking about three losses, but perhaps I would have had a less worrisome early pregnancy experience? For me the technology and advancements that have been made are one of the privileges of living in this day and age. We would be unwise not to pursue all of the opportunities available through these methods and to seek out the reassurance we would need throughout our next pregnancy journey.

Puppy Love

This last miscarriage was certainly the hardest, and I found it difficult to pick myself up and get back to normality, whatever that looked like. The fact that now every medical professional we met started to brand me as a 'recurrent miscarriage' patient, made me feel classified as a lost cause. Many times I was told that there was often no real solution to recurrent miscarriage, but to keep trying. How many times do you keep trying, I asked myself. When is enough, enough? This started to feel more real than it had ever before. The reality was that there could be something in fact wrong with me, something stopping these pregnancies, and the actuality that this may no longer be a matter of bad luck was becoming stronger.

I guess what I'm saying is that at this point I was starting to believe that our dreams of having our own baby might never be a reality. I wanted to be a mother, I knew that my heart wanted to love another little being, help it grow, nurture its learning, and with the thought that this may never be something I could provide, I ached with sadness.

My husband knew that this miscarriage had been hard both physically and emotionally, as he watched me deteriorate over those weeks in and out of hospital. I was frail and depressed and my body was shattered. I was a wreck and I was lost as to what to do now!

For many years now I had been harping on at my husband to agree to adopt a dog. As a child, I had grown up with many animals, and we always had a family dog. Dogs were always the favourite of our pets, as I loved their companionship and unconditional affection they would provide. Many a time I had argued with my husband over this, and I had sulked over many lost arguments about my desire to get a puppy. My husband never owned a dog growing up, and, always very logical in his thinking, felt that it would be more of an inconvenience to our lifestyle and living arrangements. I had continued to assure him that we would walk and exercise our dog regularly, finding the right breed for our lifestyle and invest in dog walking or day care when we were working. I had also endlessly researched different breeds, firmly maintaining that the Cavalier King Charles (the breed I was set on) would be perfectly appropriate for our small home and garden, good with children and other animals, and known to be loving, protecting and nurturing. Nonetheless, my husband wasn't a dog lover, and his view was that we would be better waiting until after we started a family. In his mind, we had to do one thing at a time. I appreciated that.

However, now, the family plans were going astray; it was a year and a half, and three pregnancies on, and no baby. I needed something, someone to nurture, I needed something to keep me going. I had always wanted a dog, and I was desperate to have something else I could invest my heart and emotions into, and I felt now was the right time.

Even if by luck, if we tried again after all this and we fell pregnant, a puppy would be at least a year old, and a lovely companion as our child or children developed. After all, I grew up with dogs as a baby, and I was confident that if we were to be lucky with a fourth pregnancy, we would want the same upbringing.

Needless to say, after everything we had been through, my husband threw caution to the wind, and agreed to a puppy. I was ecstatic, beyond excited! I felt like at least I had something certain to look forward to and I quickly started researching breeders in the area. I had a mission, I was determined to find us the right puppy, and I was all of a sudden motivated by this great and important task.

My planning set into motion as I researched breeders, reviewed new litters and started thinking about timing. Finally something I could control, and I was in my element. Within a few weeks, I found the breeder I liked, we spoke and I picked the perfect little boy puppy. I had myriad pictures from the litter, and she allowed me first choice. I chose a little ruby cavalier; he was tiny with a red collar. But to be honest, they all looked cute – I could have taken any one of them – but it was the picture she sent and his gorgeous brown eyes that clinched it for me. Other than that, I ask, how do you choose?

My husband and I were able to see our new puppy at four weeks old, but we couldn't officially pick him up and take him home until eight weeks old. We decided to call him Coco, and the breeder was local and very keen for us to start socialising with him. He was so tiny when we first met him, he fit into the palm of my hand, and as I held him close to my heart he snuggled in close and just closed his eyes. My heart melted. This little fellow was ours, and we would be responsible for him.

Don't get me wrong, I realise this gorgeous puppy was no substitution for an actual human baby of our own flesh and blood. However, it was a baby puppy, it looked up at us with its big brown eyes and it was helpless, totally reliant on us to be its new parents, to love and nurture him. I fell in love immediately and my heart was hooked. He was absolutely and undeniably adorable, and he would be all ours.

For the next four weeks, the breeder sent us daily pictures of our growing puppy, and I was able to visit him on some weekends to get time to build a connection. My focus was on the arrival of our puppy, ensuring that our house and our garden were dog friendly, and anticipating the excitement of bringing a new member of the family into our home.

A change it was, and it was exactly what we needed! The first two months were full of house training, crying at night, chewing, feeding habits, trying different sleeping arrangements, and sometimes just enjoying puppy cuddles.

Biased perhaps, but this puppy was super cute, and he was suddenly a part of our family before we knew it.

My husband, who had been apparently averse to dogs, was suddenly getting up at two a.m. to take the puppy outside for a toilet break, and I'd often find him talking to the dog and snuggling him as he watched football. It warmed my heart to see them connect so easily, and I knew immediately we had made the right decision.

It was in a sense like having a baby, although I would say the puppy is somewhat easier. Perhaps it was like baby training? For us it was all consuming, but precisely what we needed to keep our focus moving forward and not allowing us to dwell in the sad past.

A good friend, who had also experienced multiple miscarriages, said to me once that for each of her miscarriages, she and her husband found a way to move forward through 'something'. After one of their losses, they adopted a cat, another one they went away on a holiday and after their third, they bought an indulgent gift for the both of them. It was their way of helping themselves to move forward, and it reassured me that we weren't being reactive in our decision to adopt a puppy.

Our puppy was a way forward for us, and he helped us heal together as a family unit. He quickly became a very major part of our family, our lifestyle and habits and the decisions we made about everyday activities. It was incredible how important this little lovable animal became to both myself and my husband, and how each day we appreciated what he had brought into our house. As a puppy, his energy and constant playful behaviour brought back laughter and light, and his affectionate little demeanour was just what we both needed at this particular time in our lives. We may or may not finally have a baby of our own, however we knew that this little puppy would be part of our growing family if that day ever arrived.

A Good Egg

We agreed that if we wanted to continue our quest for children, we needed to find out more about what was happening before starting again. To be honest, my body had needed the break, and it was nice to just not think about cycles, fertility and testing for a while. We made an appointment with a fertility specialist just over a month after my miscarriage stopped. We really just wanted to sit down with someone who could advise us on what we should be doing next, or how we should be approaching our next pregnancy.

Until now, we hadn't really sought any professional advice; we had just gone with the natural approach and a little bit of planned timing. It wasn't a long appointment but it was helpful. Both of us underwent separate tests. There were options to do a basic level of testing and advanced. Of course the advanced level was extremely expensive and more time consuming. We just wanted the simple answers and a conversation right now, so we went for the first level of tests.

The first results of the test gave pretty straightforward answers. There isn't something immediately wrong, we can conceive and both of us have the right tools in place to get to that point. My husband was completely healthy, it transpired from all his tests, and I had a large number of egg reserves available for my age. We'd also proven this with three pregnancies in a twelve-month period.

The consultant sat down with both of us after our tests and results, and he discussed recurrent miscarriages. Again, I hadn't read much about this until my last miscarriage, as the fact that we were getting pregnant seemed to me to be the success we needed to make the whole journey. I had assumed until this last miscarriage that the first two losses were really just a bit of bad luck. Now, a pattern of three seemed to have much more serious implications.

He explained first that it could be chromosomal abnormalities. The challenge was that that the last miscarriage happened naturally, and to do this test we really needed the foetus from the miscarriage to understand if this was in fact a cause. Essentially he told us that either my husband's sperm or my eggs may not have made up enough chromosomes, or perhaps had too many to enable the foetus to develop normally. He also explained that genetic problems often lead to early miscarriage, or could cause problems for a baby when it's born. Not reassuring!

He also explained another condition often called 'sticky blood', and it's otherwise known as Hughes

Syndrome. Essentially it causes blood clots, which stop the foetus developing; after all, those little veins were less than a quarter of a millimetre at the times I had miscarried. There is a test for this, albeit quite expensive, and if it is this condition, it's treatable. He explained that if this was what I had, it could also cause preeclampsia, stillbirth or premature labour if not treated. All very daunting topics!

He said that there could be other issues such as polycystic ovaries or problems with the uterus and its shape, but we agreed that these couldn't be the problem, given that I'd had ample scans and even surgical laparoscopies over the years which had never identified these before.

The only other issue he did mention was that perhaps it was, in fact, my age. My eggs were now thirty-seven years old, and aging every day. He told us that whilst we have plenty of eggs available, it could be the quality of the eggs remaining that were the problem. Every year that I get older, my egg quality declines, and now it is just a matter of luck and chance - finding that one good egg!

Now, when we did start this pregnancy journey I didn't actually feel old. I felt like this was the right time for where we were at in life – our circumstances – and I certainly didn't think that age would be a real issue. We were healthy, energetic and could see ourselves running around after a toddler like any parent would. Now I felt like the biological clock was getting louder and louder, and the weariness of age started to loom over me. Was I really too old to have children now? Did I miss our window?

He did go on to say that many women in their early forties are still having children and that often it could take a few pregnancies to get to a quality egg, but that unfortunately for me, it may just be the endurance of continued trying. That didn't make me feel much better to be honest. He advised me that, if we were to try again I should take aspirin to help thin the blood, and he also prescribed me with some progesterone to take once we had a positive test. Both of these he said could help my body accept the pregnancy, and potentially improve the chances of the foetus developing in the very early stages. Other than that, this was all the advice he could offer right now – unless we wanted to take on some more intrusive testing. Both my husband and I agreed that we were uncertain about pursuing additional testing, and understood that in doing so we were leaving a lot to chance. Whilst that may not make sense to most, we agreed further testing at this point in time was a further reminder of the past. We desperately needed to move on and heal, and we would certainly wait a little while longer before trying again.

I have to admit I left that appointment that day feeling old and having lost a little hope of what could be. We took lots of information away, including options to understand our genetics better or whether I had sticky blood, and we decided to revisit these when we were ready. There was also information on IVF should we decide to follow that path, and even surrogacy, which both felt a little premature as options we needed to consider right now. We spoke about what next, and how we wanted to go forward from here, and we were both unanimous in our thinking. We would wait, not too long but just enough until we were both ready, and then we would try one more time, taking the additional prescription and aspirin and hope for the best. This worked for both of us, and seemed to place the least amount of pressure on us right at this point of time. Our main prerogative right now was to enjoy life with our new puppy dog, and some quality time together.

Spring is in the Air

After a terribly dim winter with constant rain and a grey outlook, spring arrived in the UK and it was beautiful! We had a lovely few months, with family visiting and some cosy romantic weekends away just my husband, our puppy and myself. I felt good again, revived, and we had time to discuss our future, looking at it from different angles with or without a family. We knew that we would try again, but the realism had started to set in that we needed to be open to other options if this didn't work out. I'm not saying it still wasn't hard, but there was an acceptance of what we had experienced, and an appreciation of what we had already, and that was a good place to be.

I would suggest that by now you know that once we start trying, it's a fairly certain conclusion that we'd be pregnant again in the following months. This was no different. Having had a couple of months' break from the entire pregnancy process, we were now relaxed. It was the first May bank holiday and we had booked the long weekend away at a dog-friendly beachside resort with our new puppy. The sun was out and it was the perfect setting for long walks, sitting outdoors with a light meal and a glass of wine, and just getting some proper British sunshine.

Lo and behold, a couple of weeks later I was holding up my pregnancy test with a positive result! My husband was a little gobsmacked, as I bounced back into bed one morning with the pregnancy test stick in my hand showing a positive result. It happened so quickly! I felt really confident this time, and I had been following the consultant's advice with my daily aspirin, and I would start taking the progesterone immediately. Whilst the progesterone was in the form of suppositories, and they weren't the most elegant of medications, needs must, and I was determined to be holding our beautiful baby that following February.

We had some lovely events planned over the spring and summer, with celebrations, holidays and days out, and I started planning which of my friends I would tell our secret to during the first trimester. I was also excited as one of my very good friends was getting married, and we had hen parties, pre-wedding celebrations and the big day, and of course I had to think about a growing tummy and what my wardrobe options could be.

I was also to be closely monitored throughout this pregnancy with my first scan booked at just over five weeks. That, in sorts, comforted me, knowing that I would have regular updates on how everything was progressing. I also felt different this time. I quickly had symptoms and some I'd never experienced in full before. My boobs were so very tender, and there was a constant pulling and stretching feeling in my lower abdomen, giving me assurance that things were moving and growing inside me. I also had bouts of nausea and constant heartburn. All good signs, I kept telling myself.

At my five-week scan I was nervous; I was back in that early pregnancy unit where everything had gone so wrong last time. My husband was travelling for work and couldn't make the appointment. I was not worried however, as I felt good, I felt pregnant. I knew that they wouldn't see much, but they did want to see me to ensure that there was a pregnancy sac visible and to get some blood tests.

The sonographer was a male this time, and to be honest his bedside manner was the worst I'd experienced so far. He conducted an internal scan as it was so early, and he did not say a word the entire time. He then bluntly told me to get dressed and take a seat beside the small desk in the same room. I followed his orders and waited. He sat at the small desk and typed with two fingers, staring intently at his computer monitor, whilst I sat beside him waiting. This went on for over ten minutes. All the time he did not speak to me. I couldn't help myself at this point, the silence was deafening.

'What did you see?' I was still anxious even though I felt more confident with this pregnancy, and this room had always made me feel so nervous, so sceptical.

'Wait a minute, I'm writing it up.' He didn't even look up as he spoke, and he continued to type awkwardly with two fingers for another twenty-five minutes. I sat there watching the clock on my iPhone just waiting. I was getting frustrated, and I was ready to give him an earful about patient empathy and compassion during these terribly nervous times. These experiences really made me question those who entered the health profession, and whether they were really best suited to roles dealing directly with patients. It took all my will to not spout out words of advice or just walk out. More so, as the time progressed, I became more and more nervous of what these results could be. He finally stopped typing and he turned to me. It had seemed like an eternity of waiting in anticipation, and his facial expression didn't even recognise the anxiety he was putting me through.

'Well, I saw something, it could be a pregnancy or it could be a cyst.' He was so nonchalant in his response, like it wouldn't matter to me either way. 'I couldn't see anything in your fallopian tubes, but I won't rule out ectopic yet, as I can't be sure what I saw in your uterus. You may want to do a blood test.' How he was still employed I had no idea; surely he didn't speak to all his patients this way?

'So should I be worried?' I asked. I was confused; he wasn't giving me anything here.

'I can't really say at this stage. You're only five weeks, so it's still early.'

'OK, so I'll have a blood test.' I had to take charge of this situation before I lost my temper, and this guy was doing nothing to help reassure me. I felt sorry for the other patients he would be consulting with that day, he was absolutely useless! He barely said much more, just directed me to another seating area where I waited for a nurse to take my bloods. I really wasn't sure what I should do next, so I just waited.

I went home after the blood tests, and reconciled with myself that he saw something, and at five weeks it was barely a quarter of a millimetre. The something he had seen was in my uterus so it was in the right place, and all things considered I'd be in for another scan by the end of the week. By then I'd be just over five and a half weeks, there should certainly be some growth by then, and I would feel much more reassured.

It was late afternoon when the early pregnancy unit phoned me on my mobile. The nurse who spoke to me told me my pregnancy blood levels were very high, extremely high for where I was in my pregnancy. She told me that the notes the sonographer took that day didn't give her a lot of assurance of what he actually saw. I rolled my eyes, and grumbled about how he had treated me and what he had said. She was empathetic and more worried about what the blood test results could mean. She was honest and said it still could be ectopic even though he hadn't seen anything in my tubes. She wanted me to come back in for further blood tests in two days.

That week I had planned a girls' day out at Ascot races, and it was a full day event starting in the early hours with a pick up from central London, and finishing well into the evening. We had a picnic bag to bring, and I had my non-alcoholic bubbly drink already chilled and ready. I really didn't want to miss out on this, and I honestly felt absolutely fine. The nurse asked me for symptoms of pain and faintness, and I told her I had none. After much convincing, she agreed that I would keep my scan appointment for the Friday, and potentially have more blood tests then if the scan was still inconclusive. It was a matter of twenty-four hour's difference, and whilst she wasn't completely sold on the plan, she was satisfied that I would be sensible and go straight to a hospital if any pain or other symptoms started.

Well, my day at the races was fabulous, the sun was shining and I felt great, glowing even. I was with two of my very close friends, and they of course guessed my news immediately when I pulled out the non-alcoholic bubbly. They were elated with the news of another pregnancy, having understood our history of loss, and were confident also that this was definitely our time. Overall it was a lovely day out, and it enabled me to relax and just enjoy myself, putting all thoughts of the scan scheduled for the following day aside.

I felt like a regular when I turned up the next morning at the early pregnancy unit. The nurses all greeted me by first name, which unnerved me. They took me straight into the little room again, and I followed the same process of undressing and settling myself on the small examining table. This time thankfully it was the female sonographer, the one who had been at most of my prior scans. She was very sensitive to my situation, and she assured me she would tell me what she saw immediately.

Good news! There was a sac, and a small foetal pole. No heartbeat yet, but it was only five and a half weeks, and the pregnancy was dating around five weeks. At that early stage we are talking under a millimetre and she assured me it was all looking positive. She advised me that no further blood test was needed, and scheduled me for a follow up scan in ten days; by then we should definitely see a heartbeat! I was over the moon; this could be the one. This had to be our rainbow baby; I was so sure of it!

Each and Every Day

In the week between our scans we went on holiday to the south of France. It was a lovely break away from it all, to get some sunshine, and to enjoy the lush French countryside with all of its amazing scenery. We hired a car, stayed in a little villa in a small provincial French village, and enjoyed the relaxation, peace and quiet. I was reaching six weeks, and I still felt queasy, hungry and generally fatigued, all very positive signs of a growing pregnancy.

We both started thinking this could actually be real, and whilst we were excited, we still held our breath waiting for that next scan, and hoping desperately to see that little flickering heartbeat. For me that was the major hurdle in these early stages of pregnancy, seeing that heartbeat, and once we were there, I felt that this first obstacle would be cleared. My pregnancies had never grown beyond six and a half weeks, and by Monday morning, when we returned from holiday and went for that scan, I would be seven weeks. It was exciting and nerve-wracking all at the same time.

The holiday flew by, and whilst we wanted it to last forever, I was also keen to get back in that small scan room again, to find out if our baby had grown and whether its heart was pumping. I was still taking aspirin daily and administering the progesterone suppositories. It had to be working!

When we returned from holiday, my husband joined me at the scan, and he stood beside me as I lay on that examining table again. Our lady sonographer greeted me with anticipation. I was sure she was as hopeful as we were. As soon as she started the scan I saw her eyes light up.

'Good news!' she breathed happily. She smiled reassuringly at me, and I felt the wind rush from my chest in a huge sigh of relief. My husband squeezed my hand and we looked at each other and just smiled deliriously.

'I can see a heartbeat,' she explained. 'It's there, the baby is still small, measuring around six to six and a half weeks.' She paused, watched my expression and added, 'I'm not worried at all.' She knew my history and she understood the fears I'd have. When she said that, I thanked her gratefully, it was the answer I needed at that point of time. It was dating small but I could see she was hopeful, and I was assured that this pregnancy was going to be viable, and it was now further along than any other pregnancy we'd had to date. I was told to come back in again in a week's time for another follow up scan. With my history they wanted to watch me closely up to the thirteen weeks. I was grateful for that, and it also gave me the opportunity to see my growing baby week by week.

I was on cloud nine that week, and I was excitedly planning the next few months. It was my close friend's hen party that weekend, and again I had arranged for the venue to stock non-alcoholic bubbly so that I wouldn't spark any questions from our curious friends. Many of the lovely ladies at the hen knew of my history, and given it was still so early, I didn't want to encourage any questions at this stage. Whilst I was so grateful to finally have a positive experience at the scan, I still remained cautious, wanting to ensure that our pregnancy continued to progress through the following weeks.

A week later, and we were back at that early pregnancy unit again for our scan. I was now just over eight weeks pregnant! This time the nerves were a lot lower, not gone altogether, but we felt assured as I was still feeling queasy and had no signs that there was anything to worry about. The same lady from the week before greeted us, and asked how we were. I told her I was feeling good in general, and she nodded at me encouragingly. I prepared for the scan, my husband stood by my side again, and we waited.

'I'm so sorry.' The sonographer's voice brought me to reality. She was so solemn, so heartfelt. I watched her face as she looked at me and then looked back at the small screen.

'It's gone?' I couldn't comprehend; it was there last week, the heartbeat. She nodded sadly, knowing that this was heart-breaking for us. No! No it couldn't be, not

156

again! That sadness, that pain, it flooded back. My husband leant over, kissing my forehead, telling me he loved me very much.

We should be used to this now, it shouldn't be so painful, but it was, it was even more so after feeling so confident, so positive about everything. Again! We were doing this again!

I dressed and sat at the small desk in the small room again. I felt like this was a cruel merry-go-round, and we could never get off it. I didn't even wait for her to give me my options this time, I knew I wanted this removed surgically; I couldn't go through another natural miscarriage. I wanted this over with immediately.

The baby had stopped growing at six weeks and three days, just after our last scan. It was another missed miscarriage, and our fourth loss.

To be fair the nurses and the hospital were this time, amazing. With my big heavy patient history, they were well aware that I needed to be booked in immediately for the surgery, as we couldn't afford for me to start miscarrying. I also wanted the pregnancy sent away for genetic testing, as this time I needed to know for sure what was causing our miscarriages.

I was told that the surgery would be late that same afternoon, that the hospital would check me in after lunch. Just enough time to go home, change, and come back. It happened quite quickly and procedurally, and I was home late that evening, tired and sore, and no longer pregnant.

It was all a bit of a blur; I could hardly talk with shock and sadness that day, in fact we both didn't speak much about it at the time, my husband and I. When we were at the hospital we played silly online board games, or just sat in silence, mourning the loss of our fourth pregnancy. I honestly had not expected this one, I truly believed we would be walking away that day with a lovely little scan photo, and news of our growing baby. Like that, in that moment, it was all gone, taken away from us again.

We took the days following off work; I needed to recover, and we needed to be together. I also needed answers; I couldn't do this again not knowing everything, and even then it was hard to fathom the thought of starting over again.

That question again, how many times do you keep trying before you stop? We talked about that a few weeks later, and truth be told, I'm not sure there is a right or wrong answer. It's like a roulette wheel, you could keep spinning and never see your numbers up, or you could just be lucky that one time. We desperately wanted that one time, and each time we felt we were putting more on the table, losing more in the process. How much were we willing to lose?

Answers Solve Nothing

In the following weeks we received letters from the hospital after the series of tests they had sent off with the foetus and pregnancy products they'd removed from me. There were no chromosomal abnormalities, it wasn't a molar pregnancy, and there was no evidence to say that there was anything wrong with the pregnancy itself.

I also signed up to a research trial. Why not, I thought! It was a new trial drug that they had been using for years on IVF patients, something that helped the woman's body accept pregnancy, rebuilding the protein that may potentially conflict with a new pregnancy. We had firmly decided that we needed answers; we needed to know what, if anything was causing these miscarriages before we moved forward. During the research trial, I would also undergo other tests, some of which may exclude me from the trial if I was to prove positive. I was to be tested for sticky blood, and also thyroid problems.

At the same time, I took a step back and reflected on our future, what might be. It was realistic to assume that we may need to stop following this path altogether, and that we may need to think about our options, a decision that we found was becoming more imminent. I knew that my emotions, my psyche couldn't cope with much more of the same. I felt as though I'd put my life on hold now for almost eighteen months, being pregnant and then not, looking forward to a due date and the arrival of a baby, and then the rug being literally pulled out from under me. I felt as though I had planned my life for the past eighteen months around a new born baby, and everything else had been given a back seat. I needed to take the control back in my life, and start really living it properly. I didn't feel resentful for the past year or so, but I did feel that I had missed out on certain opportunities and adventures because I thought 'I may just be pregnant'. Well, the reality is that I wasn't pregnant, and we were no closer to getting there right now.

The tests from the research trial came back a few weeks later, and unfortunately I wasn't accepted. They found I actually did have a condition called Hughes Syndrome, or 'sticky blood'. Whilst it would have been beneficial to be part of this research trial, it was actually more comforting to find out that there was in fact something that may be causing these miscarriages. The research doctor advised me that this condition, which is an immune disorder, causing blood clots, could actually be responsible for things like deep vein thrombosis, strokes, and heart attacks, as well as one in six cases of recurrent miscarriage.

For me it was potentially a way forward. It was an opportunity to try one more time; but this time with a real solution. I would be referred to a haematologist, I would likely have daily injections to help thin my blood, and of course I would be monitored extremely closely throughout the entire pregnancy.

It was never a guarantee but it was a hope, and we were willing to follow it, as it may just lead to our happy ending.

What Dreams May Come

With now four miscarriages, it's been difficult to look forward and predict what my hopes for a future family may be. Dealing with infertility or pregnancy loss is different for everyone, and it's difficult to say what actually makes each of us just keep going, try again just once more, hoping for that one chance for a different outcome. Mostly it's the dream of a family and the hope that one day we will have our healthy baby in our arms. That is the dream that has kept me going, kept me looking ahead, and helped me to pick myself up and try again.

We all have our different stories to tell, and we all have our dreams for the future. There were certainly times over the past year or so where it felt that they were only dreams. Dreams or wishes that would just never come true, and that I needed to find a new journey for myself, something else to aim for. The problem was that I didn't know what else I really wanted other than growing my own little family with my husband.

There is no right way to handle loss, and as human beings we are victim to our own emotions and

162

circumstances. Could I have managed things differently? Probably! There were most certainly times where I did feel all the hope I had placed on starting a family was lost. At times I wasn't sure I would recover or find a way to cope with what lay ahead of me, to just carry on as normal.

Both my husband and I have had many of these low points, and sometimes we grieved at different times, sometimes in different ways. Our plans and hopes for our future family with each loss would come crashing down so hard and so quickly, and like a broken glass, some of the smaller shards couldn't be cleaned up immediately after the fall. Weeks or months later, our bare feet would stand on them and they would cut and bleed, still causing pain, needing more time to heal.

For me in particular, there were definitely times where I found it difficult to face the future, or start thinking about 'what's next'. I sat with some friends the other night over dinner, all of them with young children of their own, some also experienced difficulty conceiving at the time. Yet for them it was an easy solution, just 'try again'. It seems easy, and I know that once my body returns to normal again and my cycles recommence, we can 'try again'. However, there is now a constant nagging voice in the back of my mind: 'What if next time doesn't work again?' The reality of our situation starts to prevail, and we need to look at our other options.

My husband openly tells me that if we cannot have children, a future with just us and our pets is also a complete future in his eyes. I am forever grateful for his support and knowledge that he loves me regardless of whether it involves children or no children. For me, it's still difficult to think of a future without a growing family, when everything I have planned for and hoped for may never come to reality. I now have this constant feeling of helplessness, that I cannot control this part of our future, and that it's out of our hands to find a way to 'fix' it. It's now up to Mother Nature, and we are held to the hands of fate. That is a difficult concept to accept.

Through it all, the hardest times for me have always been at night time, when I'm lying in bed, trying to drift off to sleep. I've always been a dreamer and a bit of a storyteller, and I enjoy materialising my future through my dreams. Sometimes I spend hours just thinking, hoping, and creating stories in a myriad of reveries before the night's slumber takes over from my active mind. Sometimes I would lie there for hours, not sleeping, but with my eyes closed, playing with my imagination and wishfully hoping for my own 'happily ever after'.

Through all the years leading up to my marriage, even before I met my husband, I would imagine what my future would be like. I would dream of a family and what it might be like to become a parent to a playful brood of children. When we were married, my dreams turned to the imaginings of our home filled with little feet, playful tones, and our lives together as parents. Each and every night my dreams would differ slightly but they would all build into little stories of a family, siblings playing together, and each building a new set of adventures. Of course I knew that these were just dreams I had made up, but in my heart I had faith and hope that these dreams would one day take shape into a reality for me and my husband.

As you can imagine, with each pregnancy my dreams would encompass all the anticipation and exciting things that I should have experienced over the months leading to the birth of our first born child. I would create pictures in my mind of becoming full and rounded with my belly, setting up a nursery, making plans leading up to my due date, and I would fantasise about those first moments when our new born baby arrived, and that moment when we could hold him or her in our arms. It possibly sounds like I'm a little out of touch with my own reality here, perhaps slightly delusional, and I was just setting myself up for a fall. However, when I was faced with all the insecurities and adversities of early pregnancy, the only thing I could do at times was to focus on what could be, staying positive, and just letting my imagination fly away with hopes for the future. It kept me positive!

With each pregnancy loss, the nights became harder, and I would start to feel restless as it became more difficult to embark on new dreams for my future. Sometimes I would lie in bed, trying to forget the past, focusing with all my energy on what could be again. I would force my mind to foresee when it could happen again, and start my imaginings with new dreams of another baby somewhere in our future.

The hardest part was that often at these times, my thoughts would torture me with just emptiness and loss, and it was difficult to create new dreams or think about the future. Going to sleep and staying asleep has always been a challenge for me, and I've often suffered bouts of insomnia through the years. It would most commonly occur when my mind was racing with uncertainty, stress or worry. The fact was that it was hard to have dreams when my sensible side was telling me that there was something wrong, something perhaps stopping us from having children, and that maybe it would never be. Negative thoughts seemed to then aggravate my sleep deprivation, and I'd often wake, remembering the devastation of our loss, feeling the emptiness of no longer being pregnant, and I'd worry. I'd get anxious about the 'what ifs'. What if I could never fall pregnant again? What if we did fall pregnant and we had another loss? What if we were never meant to be parents? Sometimes the unanswered questions would send me senseless. I'd lie awake just questioning every motive, thinking back through every experience, and trying to plan something that I had no ability to control, never really knowing what may come next for us.

The trick to it all was to not think about it, to let fate take its course, and what will be, will be. Easier said than done! For someone who loved to dream, plan and hope I had to force myself to focus on other activities besides being pregnant or having a family. I had to give myself other dreams to fancy, whether it was career, holidays, winning the lottery or other life adventures. Sometimes I'd lie there just forcing a dream to keep myself distracted, and at times it would work, even if only for a short while.

Many people I had spoken to whilst trying to conceive or after my miscarriages offered the advice that they had heard, the stories of people trying for babies for years, who then stopped thinking about it and 'bam' had a successful pregnancy. I used to wonder to myself, how do you 'stop thinking about it'? Every day, at least several times a day, I thought about it. It was a constant in my mind, and in my dreams; it was never-ending and all consuming. Unfortunately for me, it wasn't a simple light switch, I couldn't turn it off, and I couldn't block it out. What I had to do was to rely on my other thoughts and dreams, focus on the things that would divert my grief, if only for a while, and help me find a way forward.

No Rain, No Rainbow

So you're probably thinking that this story in general has been somewhat depressing, with no good news to celebrate. 'So what's the point?' you say. Well, after much reflection and thought about what has happened to date, what we experienced and life in general, I disagree.

You may think I'm a little crazy, eccentric, or just delusional, but life is good. First of all we are happily married. To have a true partner who I love, trust and can share everything and anything with is something I should be most happy and content with. My husband is someone I can see myself growing old with merrily, and I truthfully look forward to our future together and each adventure that is thrown our way.

I'm also lucky as we are both generally fit, healthy and have a good outlook on life. Look, I'm not offering to run a marathon, or climb Mount Everest, but we keep well, we look after ourselves, and we are both grateful to be in good physical shape, both in body and mind. We have a lovely home together, with our cat and our new puppy, and our house is full of love and great memories. We of course would love to build on those memories and expand our family. In what shape or form that arrives, we will be ready.

I'm also grateful for our family and friends, those who have been with us on this entire journey. We have no major quarrels with those we love, and whilst we all have our odd arguments and tiffs, we are a close knit group of family and friends. We are lucky as we enjoy our social lives and many adventures with those who are our nearest and dearest.

On top of this, my husband and I both have good solid jobs, career prospects and opportunities for a future that will provide a lifestyle we can be very content with. We have our house, and financial freedom, and we have many exciting plans and dreams for our future together. So really, I cannot groan that life has been unfair to us, and that we deserve more. I can, of course, have moments of upset or sadness, where I feel the experience itself has been unfair. But that is exactly what it is, an experience, a moment of life, something that tests us and our strength, and it is part of the ups and downs of life. It's been important for me to focus on everything in just this way, to keep myself resolute on what is great in my life, and what I needed to be grateful for. I need to think this way, to ponder on a future that could be, always keeping the hope alive.

The reality is we may never conceive naturally, we may never have our own flesh and blood baby. We may need to look at alternative options or we may need to make a decision that parenthood is not meant to be for us. These are decisions that many couples are often faced with all over the world. We are not alone, I know that. Many couples are making decisions similar to ours, sometimes harder decisions on a daily basis. The fact that we are 'relatively young' and healthy, sometimes has nothing to do with Mother Nature's decision-making process.

On the positive side, our next pregnancy may be successful; we may result in a happy, healthy rainbow baby or even multiple babies. Who knows? That's the beauty of life and what it beholds. That's the mystery that I'm excited to be a part of and why I'm excited about what happens next.

However, the decision I have made at this point is to stop thinking and just enjoy it all. When do you stop trying? As I've said before, I honestly don't know the answer right now. It's a difficult question. We know we fall pregnant, we know that's not the issue. Each time we do, we hope for the positive outcome. We haven't had luck so far, but how do you know whether next time will be the time? It's like gambling. We keep rolling the dice, hoping to come up trumps, and if we roll the dice right on the right cycle, we may just win the jackpot, our bouncy rainbow baby. But we could just keep rolling, and end up with odds. That's the name of the game I guess.

How much can my mind and my body take, as we keep rolling the dice? How many times can my husband watch me go through the highs and lows of trying, getting a pregnancy result, and then worrying through those first weeks until we hear the news of a heart beat or none? It pains him every time, and he feels helpless, yet he doesn't want to tell me to stop, as only I can know my own body's limits.

These are the quandaries we now face at this point in time. We have hope, but we have fear and experience that tells us that there is a strong possibility we may experience similar loss again and again. Each day draws new breath and new hope, as I see so many successful pregnancies around me and families growing beyond their challenges. I have to believe with all of my heart and soul that our time will come.

Over the Rainbow

Perhaps after four miscarriages, the heartache and grief, the physical strain, a number of medical investigations, and feeling at this point a little like a test guinea pig in an experimental lab, I should give up? There are certainly many options out there, adoption, fostering, or being completely content with being a fun aunty, an adoring godmother and a loving wife. These are all things that do make me complete and happy, but I also know that right now I want to give our pregnancy and family plans every opportunity to be a reality. I don't want to look back in life and wish we had tried that one more time, or given another option a chance.

In the end, if it never works, would we both be OK never having our own children? Was it all enough? It probably is, and I know we would survive it together, regardless of the outcome. Nevertheless, at this point in time I do want to try again, to be a parent in some way shape or form. For me, it's been a lifelong dream to be a mum, and above everything else, I know that both my husband and I will be loving parents. We need to give ourselves every opportunity, to give it at least one more go.

I have read so many different pregnancy stories along my journey, and many came from online forums or baby journals. There are countless women out there with so many stories of heartbreak, pain and grief, with many experiencing loss much worse than my own. Yet, it is the stories of success after so many losses that keep me hopeful for the future.

Those brave, strong ladies who have experienced as many as eight or more tragic losses at various stages of their pregnancies, those who have been trying for years and who are now are in the late stages of pregnancy or even blessed with their bouncy rainbow baby. These are the stories that keep me looking forward.

I don't have the great success story so far, but I do have a lot to be thankful for in my life, and I also pray that one day I will be lucky and blessed with a baby in the future. Today I still remain determined to continue down this path, and I understand that tomorrow that path may change its direction, and it may even get bumpier and harder to walk along, with many different obstacles to overcome. That is the beauty of life, and certainly I'm not alone in my course, I know that. I have many people walking beside me, and helping me along this journey.

Had I finished this story with a happy ending, with a successful pregnancy, it would all feel a little contrived and potentially predictable. We've all read those books, and we love them, but that's not my story today. And my story is not unfinished, it is just where it's at, within this stage of my life, and I'm content with that.

What I believe is that we all have a destiny in life, and whilst it is sometimes unfair, perhaps the challenges we have been through in trying to conceive and have a baby will help us become stronger parents in the future.

I truly have faith that our future will have a child in it, and we will find a way to become parents. What I have learnt most about what we have been through is that we are alive, we are determined, and we have kept our hope strong. In any event I have learned that remaining positive is the first step to reaching our dreams, and hopefully we will be lucky and find that rainbow one day.

My eyes are wide open now and I understand what I am getting myself into by starting all over again, both physically and emotionally. I am not saying by any means, that should we lose another baby in the process, it would be easy; I know I would experience the same loss and grief all over again. In saying that, I also know my own emotions and limits. We are ready to try again, and I know that I will always remain hopeful for what the future may bring.

The End

Thank you for reading my story.

Embracing the Storm

It's not really the end though. My last words in **Finding the Rainbow** were that we were ready to start again, and that we would remain hopeful for our future.

I'm not ready to give up this journey just yet. **Embracing the Storm** is the next chapter in my story. Even though we had finally found a potential reason for our miscarriages, and we thought it would all be smooth sailing from there on towards our baby dream. But we were being naïve.

Unfortunately we had more hurdles to face: an unexpected new medical condition, decisions about IVF, adoption or surrogacy and even the quandary of whether or not we were in fact meant to be parents. The storm continued to rumble over our heads, but we were prepared as a couple to face it head on. Like many others in our situation, our dreams of having a healthy baby made us more determined than ever to overcome any setbacks we faced.

Embracing the Storm, by *Rachel McGrath* will be available on paperback and eBook in early 2017.

BOOKS BY RACHEL McGRATH

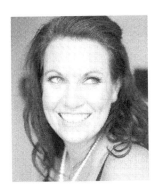

Non-Fiction, Memoir
Finding the Rainbow
Eye of the Storm
Embracing the Storm (2017)

Children's Fiction
Mud on your Face
Grimwald's Evil Plan
The Willow and Coco Children's Series

Fiction
Dark & Twisty, A Twisted Anthology
Tortured Minds
Unfinished Chapters (Contributor)

Made in the USA
San Bernardino, CA
23 May 2018